Contents

Foreword

Due to deleterious changes in the cardiovascular system associated with the ageing process cardiovascular disease is, along with cancer, the major cause of death in older individuals. As life expectancy is increasing in most developed societies, there is now an overlap between "normal" vascular ageing and "premature" vascular ageing due to a number of known, and maybe some as yet unknown, cardiovascular risk factors. Indeed, age itself should no longer be considered as a non-modifiable risk factor. This makes cardiovascular risk assessment increasingly difficult and clinicians and researchers are constantly striving to improve risk stratification in order to better deliver cost-effective screening and intervention programmes to reduce the burden of cardiovascular disease. It is encouraging that there has already been a decline in coronary artery disease mortality in the UK, and nearly 50% of this decrease can be attributed to reductions in established risk factors. Although secondary prevention strategies have been very successful in reducing mortality from cardiovascular disease, there are increasing numbers of individuals suffering from conditions such as angina, heart failure and peripheral vascular disease. It is therefore clear that our efforts should now be focused on targeting individuals at risk and offering them evidence-based treatment for the primary prevention of cardiovascular disease. This book is therefore very timely, as it sets out clearly the size of the problem and then deals with the known important individual risk factors.

Lifestyle modification is probably the most effective intervention but often gets forgotten due to the pressure to use drug intervention to reduce cardiovascular risk. The chapters on lifestyle and obesity are therefore particularly relevant and deal with evidence of the effectiveness of the main lifestyle interventions in a clear and easy to understand style. In a world where almost a third of the population are overweight, obesity is clearly a major public health problem, so it is important to emphasize, as this section does, the risk of cardiovascular disease associated with obesity and also the available therapeutic interventions.

This book also updates current knowledge on the big three risk factors, namely dyslipidaemia, diabetes and hypertension, giving clear and well set out information on evidence-based strategies for effective clinical management of these conditions.

Finally, and perhaps most importantly, there is a chapter on patient issues and compliance. In order to be most effective, any risk factor reduction programme should involve patient empowerment through education and involvement in their treatment. This chapter contains a myriad of useful tips and is followed by well set out case histories drawn from real life.

Cardiovascular Risk Management

Edited by

W. Stephen Waring BMedSci, PhD, FRCP(Ed)
Consultant Physician
Royal Infirmary of Edinburgh
Honorary Senior Lecturer
The University of Edinburgh, Edinburgh, UK

Foreword by
John Cockcroft MB ChB, FRCP
Professor of Cardiology
Wales Heart Research Institute, University Hospital Heath Park, Cardiff, UK

CHURCHILL
LIVINGSTONE

ELSEVIER

EDINBURGH   LONDON   NEW YORK   OXFORD   PHILADELPHIA   ST LOUIS   SYDNEY   TORONTO   2007

CHURCHILL LIVINGSTONE
ELSEVIER

© 2007, Elsevier Limited. All rights reserved.
Content based on a four-part series, *Risk Management in Cardiovascular Disease*, originally published in Canada. Copyright 2002–2004 Elsevier Science Ltd.

ISBN-13: 9780443101748
ISBN-10: 0443101744

British Library Cataloguing in Publication Data
A catalogue record for this book is available from the British Library

Library of Congress Cataloging in Publication Data
A catalog record for this book is available from the Library of Congress

Cover and title page image depicting the pathophysiology of systolic heart failure courtesy of Anton Becker. Cover image showing the right internal carotid artery with distal occlusion and posterior cerebral artery collaterals reproduced with permission from Hennerici M, Bogousslavsky J, Sacco R. In Clinical Practice: Stroke. Oxford: Elsevier, 2005. ©Elsevier.

Note
Knowledge and best practice in this field are constantly changing. As new research and experience broaden our knowledge, changes in practice, treatment and drug therapy may become necessary or appropriate. Readers are advised to check the most current information provided (i) on procedures featured or (ii) by the manufacturer of each product to be administered, to verify the recommended dose or formula, the method and duration of administration, and contraindications. It is the responsibility of the practitioner, relying on their own experience and knowledge of the patient, to make diagnoses, to determine dosages and the best treatment for each individual patient, and to take all appropriate safety precautions. To the fullest extent of the law, neither the Publisher nor the Authors assumes any liability for any injury and/or damage to persons or property arising out or related to any use of the material contained in this book.

The Publisher

The Publisher's policy is to use **paper manufactured from sustainable forests**

Printed in Spain

Secondary prevention has already been demonstrated to be highly effective in the reduction of vascular morbidity and mortality. However, at present, we have probably reached the limits of risk reduction in terms of secondary prevention. It is therefore primary prevention strategies based on up-to-date knowledge of cardiovascular risk that will deliver the largest reductions in cardiovascular morbidity and mortality over the next decade. This book gives a contemporary and comprehensive guide as to how such benefits can be achieved in clinical practice.

John Cockcroft
Professor of Cardiology
Wales Heart Research Institute
University Hospital Heath Park
Cardiff, UK

Preface

Over recent years, there has been increased recognition and treatment of individual risk factors for cardiovascular disease including diabetes, hypertension and hypercholesterolaemia. Nonetheless cardiovascular disease remains the leading cause of death worldwide. Despite greater public awareness, a significant proportion of children and adults regularly use tobacco and undertake insufficient physical exercise. The prevalence of obesity and type 2 diabetes is increasing rapidly, which suggests that cardiovascular disease is likely to continue to have a significant impact into the near future. While fewer people are dying prematurely from cardiovascular disease, more are living with it, and this imposes a major socioeconomic burden.

Intensive basic and clinical research has improved our understanding of mechanisms that link the presence of major risk factors with the development of cardiovascular disease, and of the significance of the interplay between these various risk factors. Historically, individual cardiovascular risk factors have been dealt with in isolation. For example, clinicians with a specialist interest in diabetes mellitus or hypertension or hypercholesterolaemia may have treated patients. Progress over the past 10 years has seen greater integration of these approaches, which better addresses overall cardiovascular risk. Clinical decision making is now directed by the patient's predicted risk, whereas previously treatment decisions had generally been based on arbitrary cut-off values for individual factors. Addressing overall risk as a target has facilitated better clinical care, and demonstrated the benefits of combining a number of different strategies to lower cardiovascular risk.

There is continued active research into the mechanisms of cardiovascular disease, and optimal preventative strategies are continually evolving. National and international clinical guidelines are frequently modified and updated, and these should be regarded as the "gold standard" to be adopted into local practice. It is hoped that this book will guide readers through some of the pertinent clinical trial data that underpin modern management of cardiovascular risk.

W. Stephen Waring
Consultant Physician
Royal Infirmary of Edinburgh
Honorary Senior Lecturer
The University of Edinburgh
Edinburgh, UK

Biography

W. Stephen Waring BMedSci, PhD, FRCP(Ed) qualified from the Queen's University of Belfast in Medicine, with a first class honours intercalated degree in Clinical Pharmacology and Therapeutics.

His general medical training was in South East Scotland, and he later worked as a Lecturer in Clinical Pharmacology for the University of Edinburgh. He was awarded a Bristol-Myers Squibb Cardiovascular Research Fellowship, and his PhD research examined links between insulin resistance syndromes, hypertension and cardiovascular risk. He has also worked as a Research Physician involved in the early development of new cardiovascular medicines within the pharmaceutical industry.

His current role is as Consultant Physician in the Royal Infirmary of Edinburgh, and honorary Senior Lecturer in the University of Edinburgh. This role involves participation in a busy Cardiovascular Risk Clinic, General Medicine duties, and a substantial interest in Clinical Toxicology.

Acknowledgement

Special thanks are deserved by Ann Stringer for her considerable assistance during the preparation of this book.

Contributors

This book is based upon the four-part series, *Risk Management in Cardiovascular Disease*, originally published in Canada. Editors and contributors to this series are as follows:

Risk Management in Cardiovascular Disease
Series Editors

Denis Drouin MD
Clinical Professor of Family Medicine; Associate Director, CME Office
Faculty of Médecine, Laval University
Québec
Canada

Peter Liu MD FRCP(C)
Director, Heart and Stroke
Richard Lewar Centre of Excellence
Toronto General Hospital
Toronto, Ontario
Canada

Volume 1. Hypertension and Other Risk Factors in Diabetes

Sheldon Tobe MD
Director, Division of Nephrology
Sunnybrook and Women's College Health Sciences Centre
Assistant Professor of Medicine
University of Toronto
Toronto, Ontario
Canada

Lawrence A. Leiter MD FRCPC FACP
Professor of Medicine & Nutritional Sciences
University of Toronto
Head, Division of Endocrinology & Metabolism
St Michael's Hospital
Toronto, Ontario
Canada

With algorithms supplied by David M.J. Naimark, Michelle Bott, Joan Basiuk and Sheldon W. Tobe.

Volume 2. Systolic Hypertension

Norman Campbell MD
Professor of Medicine, Pharmacology and Therapeutics
Department of Medicine
University of Calgary
Alberta
Canada

Volume 3. Coronary Artery Disease

G.B. John Mancini MD FRCP FACC
Professor and Head
Department of Medicine
University of British Columbia
Vancouver, BC
Canada

Volume 4. Hypertension and Lipid Disorders

Robert A. Hegele MD FRCP(C) FACP
Professor, Medicine & Biochemistry
University of Western Ontario
Endocrinologist
London Health Sciences Centre
Blackburn Scientist, Robarts Research Institute
Canada Research Chair in Human Genetics
London, Ontario
Canada

Ross Feldman MD FRCP(C)
RW Gunton Professor of Therapeutics
University of Western Ontario
Deputy Scientific Director
Robarts Research Institute
London, Ontario
Canada

Introduction
Epidemiology

Cardiovascular disease, including coronary artery disease (CAD) and stroke, remains the single leading cause of death in adults worldwide[1] and is expected to remain so well into this century.[2] The leading causes of death worldwide are shown in Figure 1.[3]

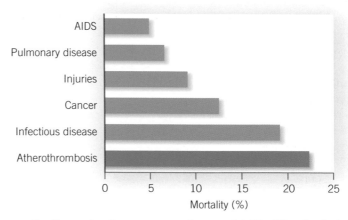

Fig. 1 Global mortality in 2002 by cause. Data from World Health Organization. The World Health Report 2004 – Changing History. Geneva: WHO, 2004.

Cardiovascular disease accounts for around 1.95 million deaths in Europe annually, and approximately 30% of deaths in patients under the age of 65 years. Between a third and a half of cardiovascular deaths are due to CAD, and about a quarter are due to stroke. The contribution of cardiovascular disease to overall mortality in Europe is shown in Figure 2.[4]

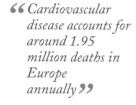

" Cardiovascular disease accounts for around 1.95 million deaths in Europe annually "

In Europe, CAD alone is responsible for 23% of deaths in women and 21% of deaths in men. Stroke by itself is the second most common cause of death in Europe, and accounts for 1.28 million deaths annually. Over one in six women (18%) and one in ten men (11%) who have had a stroke die as a complication.

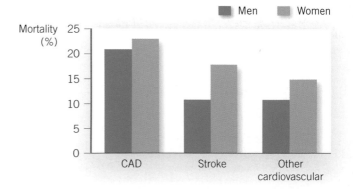

Fig. 2 Percentage of total mortality attributable to CAD, stroke and other cardiovascular disease in men and women in Europe 2003. Data from BHF Coronary heart disease statistics at www.heartstats.org

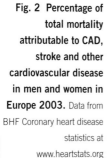

Atherosclerosis is a complex pathological process during which atheroma (lipid-filled plaques) develop within the intima of large- and medium-sized arteries, including the coronary vessels. Macrophages and vascular smooth muscle cells also accumulate within these plaques. Plaque rupture triggers platelet activation and thrombus formation, causing further luminal obstruction and reduction of blood flow. CAD, or "ischaemic heart disease" or "coronary heart disease", accounts for a significant proportion of all cardiovascular disease, and usually results from coronary obstruction due to atherosclerosis, although changes in smooth muscle tone in the coronary arteries can also be significant. In CAD there is a precarious balance between myocardial oxygen demand and supply, and a small increase in demand may precipitate acute myocardial ischaemia.

"Atherosclerosis is a complex pathological process"

CAD most commonly manifests itself as one of the following medical conditions:

- angina pectoris
- arrhythmia and sudden cardiac death
- heart failure
- coronary death
- myocardial infarction (MI).

CAD accounted for 7.2 million deaths worldwide in 1996, and by 2020 this figure is expected to have risen to more than 11 million deaths, representing a 54% increase. The lifetime risk of developing CAD at age 40 years is as high as one in two for men and one in three for women. By age 70 years lifetime risk remains as high as one in three for men and one in four for women (Figure 3).[5]

"CAD accounted for 7.2 million deaths worldwide in 1996"

Data from the UK also show cardiovascular disease to be the leading cause of mortality. In 2003, more than one in three people (38%) died from cardiovascular disease, accounting for about 233,000 deaths. Heart disease was responsible for most of the cardiovascular mortality burden (147,500 deaths), and 114,000 deaths were directly

Age (years)	Lifetime risk	
	Men	Women
40	48.6%	31.7%
50	46.9%	31.1%
60	42.7%	29.0%
70	34.9%	24.2%

Fig. 3 Lifetime risk of first CAD event.

Reproduced with permission from Lloyd-Jones DM, Larson MG, Beiser A, Levy D. Lifetime risk of developing coronary heart disease. Lancet 1999;353:89–92. ©Elsevier

attributable to CAD.[6] Around one in five men and one in six women died from the disease.

Cardiovascular disease is a major cause of premature death in the UK (before age 75 years). In 2003, cardiovascular disease led to around 65,000 premature deaths, representing 34% and 25% of premature mortality in men and women, respectively. CAD, by itself, accounts for 22% of premature deaths in men and 12% of premature deaths in women, and approximately 38,000 premature deaths in the UK overall. Stroke mortality in the UK has fallen over the last few decades.[6] However, stroke mortality rates have declined at a slower rate than previously, particularly in younger age groups. Trends in UK death rates from cardiovascular disease indicate a decline since the early 1970s (Figure 4).[7]

« Cardiovascular disease is a major cause of premature death in the UK »

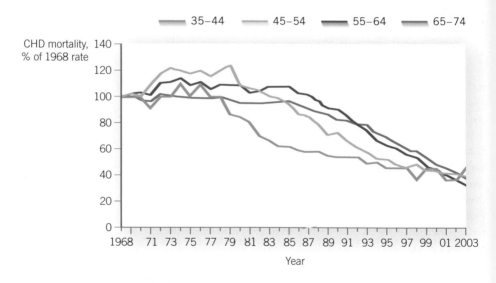

Fig. 4 **Age specific death rates from CAD in men, 1968–2003, UK, plotted as a percentage of the rate in 1968.**[7]

Data from BHF Coronary heart disease statistics at www.heartstats.org

A recent study aimed to explain the decline in mortality from CAD in the UK between 1981 and 2000. The researchers concluded that more than half (58%) of the decline in CAD mortality was attributable to reductions in major risk factors, principally smoking. Treatment of individuals, including secondary prevention, was thought to explain the remaining two-fifths (42%) of the mortality decline.[8] A similar decline in CAD mortality has been observed in the USA over the past 40 years.[9] This has been attributed to successful implementation of primary prevention programmes (25% of the decline), secondary prevention measures (29% of the decline), and better treatment of established CAD (46%).[10]

Mortality rates differ between countries, and while they have generally been declining in Westernized nations, they have continued to rise in Eastern Europe, Russia, and many developing countries.[11] The scale of these differences is exemplified by the 10-fold increase in cardiovascular disease mortality seen in Central and Eastern Europe compared with Western Europe. In Croatia, for example, deaths from CAD have risen by 60% from 1988 to 1998.[11] These alarming increases are thought to reflect underlying trends towards an increased prevalence of obesity associated with Western diets and increasing tobacco use. Given these current trends, it seems likely that the rate of CAD in "high risk" countries will continue to rise, and this threatens to pose a major cardiovascular healthcare burden for the near future.

"While mortality from CAD has tended to decline over recent years, the prevalence of CAD has been escalating"

While mortality from CAD has tended to decline over recent years, the prevalence of CAD has been escalating. This is due to a combination of factors:

- growing numbers of people surviving into advanced age
- increasing prevalence of certain risk factors (e.g. type 2 diabetes)
- improved CAD treatment and survival rates.

Therefore, despite existing efforts to implement prevention strategies to combat the key risk factors, CAD remains highly prevalent among the adult population of Westernized countries. CAD leads to health problems that will inevitably require inpatient care.

In 1999 the World Health Organization (WHO) published the findings of a 10-year study to monitor trends and determinants in cardio-vascular disease, called the MONICA project.[12] This study prospectively assessed non-fatal MI and coronary deaths in men and women from 37 populations across 21 countries, including a number of European countries; a full description of the objectives and abridged protocol is available electronically.[13] The aim was to determine trends in mortality, separating changes in coronary event rates from changes in survival. During 371 population-years, 166,000 events were reported. Results revealed a small but significant decline in the incidence of coronary disease for people of both sexes and all age groups in most Western countries studied. The MONICA project also found that in populations in which mortality had decreased, reduction in coronary event rates had contributed two thirds to this phenomenon and case fatality one third. Therefore, the MONICA project concluded that the major determinant of improvements in cardiovascular mortality was the underlying change in coronary event rates. Furthermore, this has been largely attributed to mod-ification of major cardiovascular risk factors.[14] Only hypertension, total blood cholesterol, and tobacco smoking were measured in the majority of the MONICA study participants, whereas high-density lipoprotein (HDL)-cholesterol and diabetes were not included in the core study.

"The MONICA project concluded that the major determinant of improvements in cardiovascular mortality was the underlying change in coronary event rates"

Morbidity

The true impact of cardiovascular disease on morbidity is hard to quantify. CAD causes illness and disability that limit social and economic activities, which has a major impact on quality of life for patients and can have a massive impact on the economy of populations. It should also be remembered that this affects not only the patient, but also his/her partner and other family members. Chest pain, or the fear of provoking it, may curtail numerous activities from leisure and sports, to more mundane pursuits like housework or shopping.

Some men may be reluctant to have sexual intercourse, which may then harm their personal relationships. In severe cases people might become virtually housebound and lose all social contact. Employment can also suffer, with a significant proportion of patients losing their ability to work.

❝ CAD causes illness and disability that limit social and economic activities ❞

Financial impact

Data from the WHO show that CAD is the leading cause of premature death among adults. In addition patients with established CAD require long-term medical care in the community and the consequent morbidity represents a significant health problem as well as imposing a substantial economic burden. Cardiovascular disease has been estimated to account for about 15% of healthcare delivery costs in Westernized countries, making it the single most expensive disease category. The long-term disability and illness that often results from CAD places an enormous burden on patients, their families, and healthcare providers alike.

❝ Patients with established CAD require long-term medical care in the community ❞

In 2003 productivity losses arising from cardiovascular disease mortality and morbidity were estimated to cost the UK more than £6200 million, with around 60% of this cost (£3677 million) due to death and 40% (£2556 million) due to illness in those of working age. The cost of informal care for people with cardiovascular disease in the UK was over £4800 million in 2003 (Figure 5).[4] Production losses due to mortality and morbidity associated with CAD cost the UK over £3100 million in 2003, with about 70% of this cost (£2173 million) due to death and 30% (£961 million) due to illness in those of working age. The cost of informal care for people with CAD in the UK was estimated to be £1250 million.

❝ Cardiovascular disease is estimated to cost the UK economy just under £26 billion a year ❞

Overall cardiovascular disease is estimated to cost the UK economy just under £26 billion a year. This represents an overall cost per capita of £434. Of the total cost of cardiovascular disease to the UK, approximately 57% is due to direct healthcare costs, 24% to productivity losses, and 19% to the informal care of people with cardiovascular disease (Figure 5). Overall CAD is estimated to cost the UK economy over £7.9 billion a year. This represents an overall cost

	£ million	% of total
Healthcare costs	14,732	57
Production losses due to mortality	3,677	14
Production losses due to morbidity	2,556	10
Informal care	4,835	19
Total	**25,800**	**100**

Fig. 5 Estimated economic burden of cardiovascular disease in the UK, 2003.[4] Data from BHF Coronary heart disease statistics at www.heartstats.org

per capita of £133. Of the total cost of CAD to the UK, around 45% is due to direct healthcare costs, 40% to productivity losses, and 16% to the informal care of people with CAD.

There are important financial considerations in the provision of healthcare resources for the complications of established CAD, given that survival among this population is progressively increasing. For example, year 2000 data from the UK estimate direct healthcare costs associated with post-MI congestive heart failure to be between £313–453 million annually (about 1% of total national healthcare spending), and an additional £68 million for nursing home costs. The financial implications of this one complication alone illustrate how CAD exerts a dramatic impact on direct and indirect healthcare costs in the UK.[15]

A similarly dramatic economic impact of cardiovascular disease has also been reported in the USA (Figure 6).[16]

Indirect costs associated with CAD include mortality and disability (long term and short term). Hospital care and premature mortality account for the highest costs in each category, respectively. Cardiovascular diseases represent the most expensive cost category in terms of hospital care and are the largest contributors to prescription drug costs. CAD accounts for approximately 30% of cardiovascular disease costs for each of these categories (Figure 7).

CAD exerts a dramatic impact on direct and indirect healthcare costs in the UK

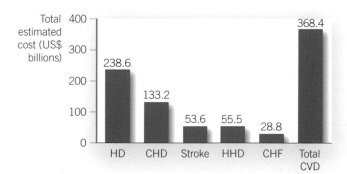

Total estimated cost (US$ billions)

- HD: 238.6
- CHD: 133.2
- Stroke: 53.6
- HHD: 55.5
- CHF: 28.8
- Total CVD: 368.4

Fig. 6 Estimated total (direct and indirect) cost of cardiovascular disease in the USA for 2003.[16] CHF = congestive heart failure; CVD = cardiovascular disease; HD = heart disease; HHD = hypertensive heart disease. Data from ref 16.

15

Fig. 7 Breakdown of direct NHS spending on cardiovascular disease in the UK, 2003.[4] A&E = Accident & Emergency department. Data from BHF Coronary heart disease statistics at www.heartstats.org

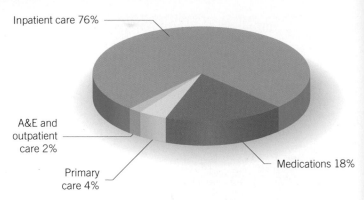

Inpatient care 76%

A&E and outpatient care 2%

Primary care 4%

Medications 18%

Cardiovascular disease prevention

It has been estimated that more than 80% of all CAD cases could be prevented if the population adhered to basic behavioural guidelines, such as regular exercise, weight control, healthy diet, not smoking, and moderate alcohol consumption.[17] In reality, however, preventing CAD is not straightforward and requires intervention on many levels, including:

- identification and treatment of risk factors (primary prevention)
- early diagnosis and optimal treatment (secondary prevention)
- limiting progression of established disease (tertiary prevention).

> *66 80% of all CAD cases could be prevented if the population adhered to basic behavioural guidelines 99*

Risk factors for cardiovascular disease

The INTERHEART study showed that nine potentially modifiable risk factors account for over 90% of the risk of an initial acute MI.[18] In decreasing order of population attributable risk these factors are: dyslipidaemia, smoking, psychosocial factors, abdominal obesity, hypertension, fruit and vegetable consumption, physical exercise, diabetes and alcohol consumption (Figure 8).

Coronary risk factors vary between men and women, between different age groups, and between those living in different socioeconomic environments. Despite greater public awareness of the detrimental health impact, the prevalence of smoking and obesity have actually increased in recent years,[19] particularly in younger people. This alarming trend signals a potential for even further increases in the burden posed by CAD in the future. In addition to the established major risk factors, recent publications have revealed several new potential targets in the prevention of CAD, such as infectious agents, inflammatory markers and micronutrients.

> *66 The prevalence of smoking and obesity have actually increased in recent years 99*

Multiple cardiovascular risk factors

The risk of CAD and stroke increases as the number of risk factors present in an individual increase (Figure 9).[20]

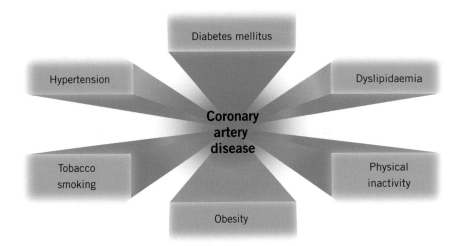

Hypertension and dyslipidaemia increase the risk of cardiovascular disease, and the presence of both risk factors further increases risk. The Framingham study was one of the first and most important epidemiological studies that defined the major CAD risk factors.[21] The investigators found that cigarette smoking, hypertension, high total cholesterol and low-density lipoprotein (LDL)-cholesterol, low HDL-cholesterol, and diabetes increased the risk of CAD, and that these risk factors were additive. An individual with a number of modest abnormalities in risk factors may be at considerably higher risk than another person with just one highly abnormal risk factor. As a result of these findings the concept of an integrated and comprehensive approach to CAD risk assessment and management has been introduced.[22]

Data from the MRFIT trial (n=347,978) support the idea that multiple risk factors, including systolic blood pressure >120 mmHg, and total cholesterol >5.2 mmol/L, independently predict cardiovascular disease mortality. Compared with a cholesterol level <5.2 mmol/L, a level >6.2 mmol/L doubled the CAD risk.[23,24] The presence of hypertension, indicated by systolic blood pressure >140 mmHg, increased the CAD risk by about 2.5 times.[25] The presence of both risk factors is at least additive and possibly synergistic. Thus, the CAD risk for an individual with both elevated blood pressure and elevated cholesterol is four to five times that of an individual without either of these major risk factors.

Risk increases with increasing number of risk factors and is even higher for a patient with diabetes or known CAD.[26] The 7-year risks of MI in subjects without diabetes with and without prior MI were 18.8% and 3.5%, respectively, while in subjects with diabetes with and without prior MI they were 45.0% and 20.2%, respectively.[26] The

Fig. 8 Major risk factors for cardiovascular disease.

"An individual with a number of modest abnormalities in risk factors may be at considerably higher risk than another person with just one highly abnormal risk factor"

17

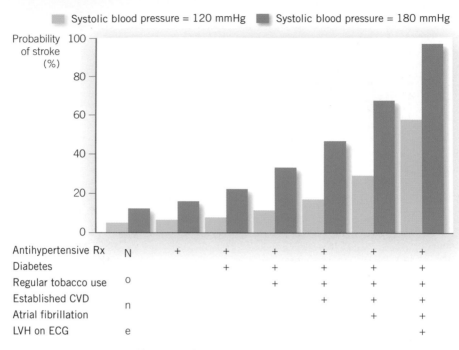

Legend: ▮ Systolic blood pressure = 120 mmHg   ▮ Systolic blood pressure = 180 mmHg

Antihypertensive Rx	N	+	+	+	+	+	+
Diabetes			+	+	+	+	+
Regular tobacco use	o			+	+	+	+
Established CVD					+	+	+
Atrial fibrillation	n					+	+
LVH on ECG	e						+

Fig. 9 The additive and synergistic effect of multiple cardiovascular risk factors on stroke risk. CVD = cardiovascular disease; LVH on ECG = voltage criteria for left ventricular hypertrophy on electrocardiogram. Reproduced with permission from Wolf PA. Prevention of stroke. Lancet 1998;352 Suppl 3:SIII15–18. ©Elsevier

effect on cardiovascular risk of having both risk factors is therefore additive and possibly synergistic.

Clustering of risk factors and metabolic syndrome

It has been observed that hypertension is commonly associated with other risk factors such as insulin resistance, obesity, hyperuricaemia, and dyslipidaemia. About 90% of patients with hypertension have at least one additional major cardiovascular risk factor, as many as 40% have two additional risk factors, and 11% have three or more.[27] The prevalence of multiple major cardiovascular risk factors in young adults is shown in Figure 10, and the prevalence in older adults is likely to be even higher.[28] Overall, the prevalence of dyslipidaemia is around 22.5–24.4% in hypertensive men and 26.3–28.6% in hypertensive women aged 35–64 years, compared with only 17.2–18.6% in men and 12.8–18.5% in women who are non-hypertensive.[29] The cluster of several cardiovascular risk factors, especially in individuals with hypertension, increases the relative risk of cardiovascular disease.[21]

The non-random association between elevated blood pressure and dyslipidaemia in the same individual has been noted for at least two decades.[30,31] An unexpectedly high prevalence of both hypertension and dyslipidaemia in young adults was noted to occur in clusters of siblings, and was labelled "familial dyslipidaemic hypertension".[32] At

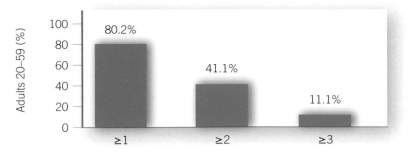

around the same time, the clustering of hypertension, obesity, diabetes and dyslipidaemia was described by Reaven – the "metabolic syndrome".[33] National survey data from the USA suggest that metabolic syndrome affects as many as 24% of adults, and prevalence is as high as 35% in men with hypertension.[34]

Fig. 10 Prevalence of multiple major cardiovascular risk factors in young adults.[250]

Obesity, in the context of endogenous and exogenous susceptibility factors, is considered to be a major aetiological factor for insulin resistance and hyperinsulinaemia and, in the context of other metabolic abnormalities, is thought to be a major risk factor for cardiovascular disease.[35,36] Insulin resistance affects a wide range of metabolically active tissues, such as skeletal muscle, adipose tissue, and the liver. The WHO and the European Group for the Study of Insulin Resistance (EGSIR) have proposed clinical definitions for the insulin resistance syndrome.[37,38]

The definition proposed by the WHO group involves measurement of insulin resistance by glucose clamp methods, which are not readily available outside dedicated clinical research facilities. The EGSIR recommend measurement of fasting insulin and glucose concentrations as surrogate markers of insulin resistance and impaired glucose tolerance (IGT), respectively, so that screening and diagnosis can be undertaken more readily in clinical practice (Figure 11). An established diagnosis of insulin resistance syndrome, using these strict criteria, predicts the subsequent development of type 2 diabetes and indicates an increased risk of cardiovascular mortality.[39,40]

Obesity is considered to be a major aetiological factor for insulin resistance and hyperinsulinaemia and is thought to be a major risk factor for cardiovascular disease

Recently the International Diabetes Federation (IDF) have produced a more user-friendly definition of metabolic syndrome with abdominal obesity, defined by waist circumference and adjusted for ethnicity, as the core feature.[41] Waist circumference is independently associated with insulin resistance, as well as hypertension and dyslipidaemia, and abdominal obesity is acknowledged as an important causative factor in metabolic syndrome. Removal of the need to establish insulin resistance in order to recognize metabolic syndrome

19

	WHO definition[37]	EGSIR definition[38]	IDF definition[41]
Mandatory:	Impaired glucose tolerance, OR type 2 diabetes, OR top quartile of insulin resistance using euglycaemic clamp	Top quartile of fasting insulin concentration, OR top quartile of insulin resistance using euglycaemic clamp	Central obesity – waist circumference ≥94 cm for Europid men and ≥80 cm for Europid women, with ethnicity specific values for other groups
Plus at least 2 of:	• Waist-hip ratio >0.9 or BMI >30 kg/m^2 • Plasma triglycerides >1.7 mmol/L • Plasma HDL cholesterol <0.9 mmol/L • Hypertension >160/90 mmHg • Microalbuminuria	• Waist circumference >94 cm (men), >80 cm (women) • Plasma triglycerides >2.0 mmol/L (or treated) • Plasma HDL cholesterol <1.0 mmol/L • Hypertension >140/90 mmHg (or treated)	• Triglycerides ≥1.7 mmol/L (or treated) • HDL <1.03 mmol/L in males or <1.29 mmol/L in females (or treated) • Hypertension systolic ≥130 mmHg or diastolic ≥85 mmHg (or treated) • Fasting plasma glucose ≥5.6 mmol/L (or diagnosed type 2 diabetes)

Fig. 11 Comparisons of WHO, IDF and EGSIR definitions of the metabolic syndrome.[37,38,41]

should increase recognition and promote intensive cardiovascular risk reduction. Importantly, by placing emphasis on abdominal obesity this definition should encourage the investigation of cardiovascular risk factors in obese patients; abdominal obesity is easily identifiable!

Similarly, the National Cholesterol Education Program (NCEP) guidelines for defining insulin resistance syndrome have incorporated readily available measurements that avoid the need for euglycaemic clamp techniques.[42]

Insulin resistance and atherosclerosis

66 *Waist circumference is independently associated with insulin resistance, as well as hypertension and dyslipidaemia* 99

The mechanistic basis of atherosclerosis in insulin resistance is multi-faceted, and includes hyperinsulinaemia and other biochemical disturbances, such as elevated plasminogen activator inhibitor-1 (PAI-1), elevated markers of inflammation, e.g. C-reactive protein (CRP), and alterations in adipocyte hormones, e.g. depressed adiponectin and elevated leptin.[43–46] The atherosclerosis risk factors that cluster together in the metabolic syndrome are shown in Figure 12. Hypertension and dyslipidaemia are fundamental components of the insulin resistance syndrome, and their relationship is complex and interdependent. For example, hyperinsulinaemia is able to directly impair vascular function, which may result in increased systemic blood pressure.[47] Hyperinsulinaemia partly compensates for insulin resistance to maintain glucose homeostasis but probably favours the pro-hypertensive effects of insulin through cellular signalling pathways. Also, insulin resistance has a profound influence on lipoprotein metabolism, and is likely to promote development of dyslipidaemia.[48] Finally, dyslipidaemia itself, in the absence of insulin resistance, can affect vascular endothelial function, which may have some regulatory implications for haemodynamics and blood pressure.[49] Thus, the relationship between elevated blood pressure and dyslipidaemia is complex, and the observed mechanistic inter-relatedness suggests that appropriate management of these clinical disturbances could have synergistic beneficial consequences ultimately resulting in reduced clinical endpoints of atherosclerosis.

Observational data generally suggest if major cardiovascular risk factors co-exist, such as hypertension and dyslipidaemia, then there is generally a multiplicative effect on the risk of CAD events. A promising finding from subgroup analyses of large statin trials is that the relative cardiovascular risk reduction seen with lipid-lowering is similar among those with high and normal blood pressure, suggesting that the beneficial effects of cholesterol lowering and blood pressure lowering are independent, and likely to be additive or synergistic.[50–54]

"Observational data generally suggest if major cardiovascular risk factors co-exist then there is generally a multiplicative effect on the risk of CAD events"

Overall cardiovascular risk prediction
Overall assessment of CAD risk incorporates combinations of the various risk factor variables, including age, sex, weight, systolic blood

Fig. 12 Atherosclerosis risk factors that cluster in the metabolic syndrome.

Atherogenic dyslipidaemia
- elevated triglycerides (>2.0 mmol/L)
- elevated LDL cholesterol (see targets for age)
- small dense LDL particles
- depressed HDL cholesterol (<0.9 mmol/L in men; <1.0 mmol/L in women)

High-normal blood pressure (>130/>85 mmHg)

Insulin resistance ± impaired fasting glucose (6.1 to 7.0 mmol/L)

Proinflammatory state indicated by more than one of:
- elevated high-sensitivity C-reactive protein (hsCRP)
- elevated homocysteine
- elevated Lipoprotein (a)

Prothrombotic state indicated by more than one of:
- elevated plasminogen activator inhibitor-1 (PAI-1)
- elevated fibrinogen
- presence of clotting factor V Leiden

> 66 *The beneficial effects of cholesterol lowering and blood pressure lowering are independent, and likely to be additive or synergistic* 99

pressure, diastolic blood pressure, blood glucose, blood lipid ratios, and smoking history. Most assess risk over a 5- or 10-year interval and are derived using equations from large population studies, e.g. the Framingham,[55] Sheffield[56] and New Zealand[57] cohorts.

A collection of commonly used clinical algorithms for cardiovascular and CAD risk prediction can be found in electronic format, for example the "Cardiovascular Risk Calculator" hosted by the University of Edinburgh,[58] and can be used as the basis for primary or secondary prevention strategies. Alternatively, the GRACE risk predictor can be used for patients who have presented with a MI or unstable angina.[59,60] A variety of other internet-based risk assessment tools are available, for example from the Medical Algorithm website at http://www.medal.org/.

Recently, the European Society for Cardiology (ESC) released the SCORE project, which is an effort to enhance accuracy by adapting the cardiovascular risk calculation to regional statistics of cardiovascular mortality (Figure 13).[61]

Similar risk scoring systems for cardiovascular disease risk have been incorporated into the updated Joint British Societies guidelines for cardiovascular risk reduction (JBS-2), as shown in Figure 14.[62] It is assumed that patients with diabetes are already at sufficiently high cardiovascular risk that calculation is not necessary, so the charts are concerned with men and women without diabetes. Similarly, those with established atherosclerotic disease (previous MI, ischaemic stroke, peripheral vascular disease, etc) are also automatically considered to be high risk, and full preventive intervention should be implemented.

> 66 *Those with established atherosclerotic disease are automatically considered to be high risk, and full preventive intervention should be implemented* 99

Such charts and algorithms help identify those individuals at risk of CAD and to determine benefits they might be likely to derive from interventions such as smoking cessation, blood pressure lowering, reducing serum cholesterol concentrations, or combinations of these. However, they should not be used as sole treatment guides.

Screening assessment

Screening for CAD risk factors should be carried out, particularly in at-risk groups (e.g. family history of CAD, smokers, obese people, the elderly), and should include measurement of blood pressure, blood glucose level and blood lipid profile.

Measurement of blood pressure is often performed inaccurately, and requires adequate patient preparation, appropriate technique, and suitable equipment. When carried out correctly, blood pressure measurement takes around 8 minutes to complete.[63]

Certain individuals are at increased risk of type 2 diabetes, and should be considered for screening for diabetes:

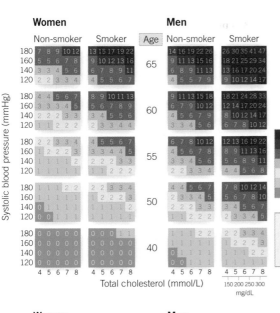

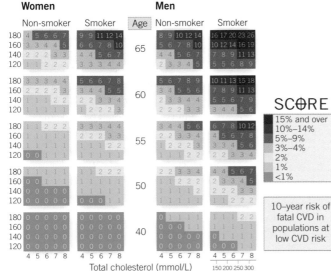

Fig. 13 10-year risk of fatal cardiovascular disease in "high" and "low" risk European populations, based on the ESC SCORE system. Reproduced with permission from Conroy RM, Pyörälä AP, Fitzgerald AP. Estimation of ten-year risk of fatal cardiovascular disease in Europe: the SCORE project. European Heart Journal 2003;24:987–1003. ©European Society of Cardiology

Screening for CAD risk factors should be carried out, and should include measurement of blood pressure, blood glucose level and blood lipid profile

- age >45 years (men and women)
- obesity (particularly abdominal)
- family history of type 2 diabetes
- known hypertension or dyslipidaemia
- physical inactivity
- gestational obesity or birth of large baby (>4.5 kg).

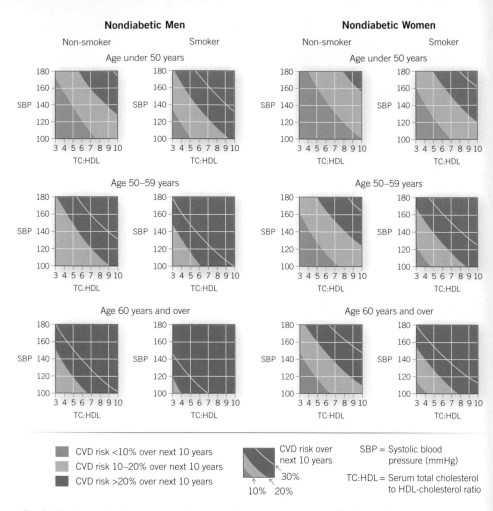

Fig. 14 Cardiovascular disease prediction charts in men and women, stratified by smoking status, age group, systolic blood pressure and total:HDL cholesterol ratio. Reproduced with permission from Joint British Societies. JBS 2: Joint British Societies' guidelines on prevention of cardiovascular disease in clinical practice. Heart 2005;91 Suppl 5:v1–52.
©BMJ Publishing Group

Patients with established atherosclerosis

There is a strong positive association between established atherosclerosis and the risk of future cardiovascular morbidity and mortality. For example, the extent of atherosclerosis affecting the carotid arteries is associated with an increased risk of cardiovascular events, and inversely associated with event-free survival (Figure 15).[64]

Similar findings have been reported for patients with established peripheral artery disease affecting the lower limbs. The severity of

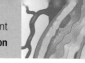

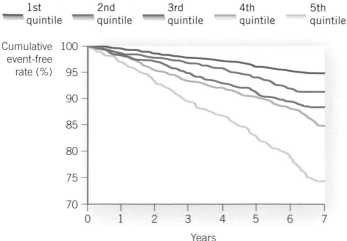

Fig. 15 **Carotid disease as a marker of cardiovascular risk.** Patients with the most extensive carotid atherosclerosis (5th quintile) had the highest risk of cardiovascular events (lowest "event-free" survival), n=4476, and the estimated cumulative combined endpoint rate for the fifth quintile was >25% at 7 years compared with <5% for the first quintile. Reproduced with permission from O'Leary DH, Polak JF, Kronmal RA, et al. Carotid-artery intima and media thickness as a risk factor for myocardial infarction and stroke in older adults. Cardiovascular Health Study Collaborative Research Group. N Engl J Med 1999;340(1):14–22. ©Massachusetts Medical Society

"The extent of atherosclerosis affecting the carotid arteries is associated with an increased risk of cardiovascular events"

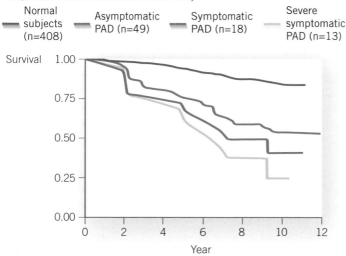

Fig. 16 **Kaplan-Meier survival curves in patients with peripheral artery disease of varying severity and healthy controls.** Peripheral arterial disease is associated with higher mortality, and there is an inverse relationship between disease severity and survival. Reproduced with permission from Criqui MH, Langer RD, Fronek A, et al. Mortality over a period of 10 years in patients with peripheral arterial disease. N Engl J Med 1992;326(6):381–386. ©Massachusetts Medical Society

Type of angina	Provocation factors	Other features
Classical	Physical exertion, cold weather, extreme emotion	Pain fades quickly with rest; pain relatively predictable
Decubitus	Occurs on lying down; commonly associated with left ventricular dysfunction	Associated with severe CAD
Nocturnal	Occurs at night, may wake patient from sleep (especially during vivid dreams)	Occurs with severe CAD disease; vasospasm may also occur
Variant (or Prinzmetal's)	Occurs without provocation, usually at rest	Associated with coronary artery spasm; more common in women
Cardiac syndrome X	Good history of angina + positive exercise ECG test + normal coronary arteries	Functional abnormalities of coronary microcirculation; more common in women
Unstable	Recent onset (<1 month), worsening angina ± at rest	Medical emergency; 10% progress to MI if untreated; 5–15% mortality within 1 year

Fig. 17 Clinical patterns of angina.

peripheral arterial disease is positively associated with cardiovascular mortality, and inversely correlated with cardiovascular disease-free survival (Figure 16).[65]

Angina pectoris is normally diagnosed on the basis of a consistent clinical history and can manifest as central or retrosternal chest discomfort described as a "heavy", "tight", "gripping" or "aching" sensation. There may also be radiation down either or both arms into the neck and jaw or upper abdomen and back. The degree of discomfort can range from a mild ache to a severe pain associated with sweating, breathlessness, nausea and vomiting. Classic provocation factors include physical exertion (particularly after meals), cold weather, and extreme anger, excitement, or other emotion (Figure 17).

The investigations normally considered helpful in patients with angina are shown in Figure 18.

In contrast, many patients with subclinical atherosclerosis are asymptomatic and finding reliable and accurate markers of occult CAD, peripheral vascular disease and cerebrovascular disease has been difficult. However, a number of non-invasive imaging techniques are available to measure and monitor atherosclerosis in asymptomatic individuals, including exercise ECG testing, computerized

❝ Many patients with subclinical atherosclerosis are asymptomatic ❞

Investigation	Details
Resting ECG	Attack shows transient ST↓ ± T-wave inversion or upright T-waves; evidence of old MI, LVH, or LBBB may be present
Exercise ECG	Positive = ST↓ >1 mm during physical exertion (particularly if chest pain occurs simultaneously); 75% patients with significant CAD will test positive
Cardiac scintigraphy	Myocardial perfusion scanning using contrast agents (at rest and post-stress)
Echocardiography	Assessment of ventricular function and ventricular wall involvement
Coronary angiography	Usually performed to delineate exact coronary anatomy in patients undergoing procedures such as CABG

tomography, magnetic resonance coronary angiography, positron emission tomography, and echocardiography. Each of these possesses relative strengths and weaknesses. Measurement of ankle to brachial systolic blood pressure (called the ankle–brachial pressure index) has also shown some promise as an early marker of atherosclerosis. The technique involves the use of a portable Doppler probe to detect pedal pulses, and a sphygmomanometer with inflatable cuff for placement around the ankle. The ankle–brachial pressure index is quick to measure, is reproducible, and is applicable to most individuals. The ankle–brachial pressure index is inversely related to measures of generalized atherosclerosis, including the prevalence of angina, previously diagnosed MI, and stroke, and a cut-off value of 0.9 or less is >90% sensitive and specific for detection of angiographically definable atherosclerosis affecting large arteries.[66] Furthermore, ankle–brachial pressure index values <0.9 are associated with a markedly increased risk of mortality and major cardiovascular events.[67]

Fig. 18 Investigations for angina pectoris.
CABG = coronary artery bypass graft; LBBB = left bundle branch block; LVH = left ventricular hypertrophy; ST↓ = ST-segment depression.

Women
CAD is commonly perceived as a disease mainly affecting men. However a similar or greater proportion of women in Europe die from CAD compared with men, and future projections predict a marked increase in female CAD mortality. Sex-specific differences arise in the clinical manifestation of cardiovascular disease, and differences in the prevalence of major risk factors for atherosclerosis. Due to the apparent protective effects of oestrogens, women tend to present with symptomatic CAD approximately 10 years later than their male counterparts.[68] Low HDL-cholesterol, raised triglyceride levels, and

❝Sex-specific differences arise in the clinical manifestation of cardiovascular disease ❞

diabetes appear to have a greater impact on increasing CAD risk in women than in men.[69]

Until recently, the role of hormone replacement therapy (HRT) in reducing CAD risk in post-menopausal women was uncertain. Observational data had suggested that HRT might decrease the frequency of CAD events in healthy post-menopausal women.[70–73] However, the results of the Women's Health Initiative (WHI) trial suggest otherwise. WHI was the first randomized controlled trial to directly address the effect of combined oestrogen plus progesterone on CAD in predominantly healthy post-menopausal women.[74] Data collected from more than 16,600 study participants showed that oestrogen plus progesterone does not confer benefit for preventing CAD among healthy women with a uterus. The Heart and Estrogen/progestin Replacement Study (HERS) was another randomized trial comparing the same regimen of oestrogen plus progestogen versus placebo, this time among 2700 women (with a uterus) with documented CAD.[75] Analysis of results indicated that HRT conferred an initial elevation in CAD risk among women with prior CAD.

> *The lifetime risk of a 50-year-old woman developing CAD is nearly three times greater than her risk of developing breast cancer*

The lifetime risk of a 50-year-old woman developing CAD is nearly three times greater than her risk of developing breast cancer, 31.1% CAD versus 11.3% breast cancer.[5] The continuing lifetime risk of CAD in women should provide an adequate rationale for aggressive screening and management of hypertension and dyslipidaemia.

> *Public health initiatives need to actively promote healthy diet, regular aerobic exercise and non-smoking behaviour in young people*

Young people

It is now known that risk behaviours for CAD and the accompanying pathophysiological vascular changes begin early in childhood. The Bogalusa Heart Study gathered cardiovascular risk data on more than 10,000 infants, children and young adults over a 25-year period.[76–78] Results showed increasing prevalence of obesity in children accompanied by raised blood pressure, adverse changes in serum lipids, and hyperinsulinaemia. Tobacco smoking during childhood was also a risk factor. Autopsy studies in young adults have found a strong association between clinical risk factors and post-mortem evidence of CAD; even the youngest children examined (aged 15 years) showed signs of coronary atheroma.[79–81] Public health initiatives need to actively promote healthy diet, regular aerobic exercise and non-smoking behaviour in young people in order to delay the progressive development of atherosclerotic disease that may present in early adulthood.

> *Screening and management of major CAD risk factors should be pursued in the elderly*

Elderly patients

Clinicians are often more reluctant to treat older patients at risk from CAD than younger ones, despite the knowledge that treating isolated systolic hypertension (ISH) and hypercholesterolaemia in the elderly decreases the frequency of CAD events and stroke.[82–86] As for women, screening and management of these major CAD risk factors should be pursued in the elderly.

Summary

Cardiovascular disease is the leading cause of death and illness in Europe, as well as in the rest of the world. A large proportion of this mortality and morbidity is represented by CAD. Despite the observation that early mortality from cardiovascular disease is falling, the prevalence of heart disease and stroke is reaching almost epidemic proportions. Due to the rising numbers of elderly people in the population and adverse changes in lifestyle, this proliferation is set to continue well into the 21st century.

"The prevalence of heart disease and stroke is reaching almost epidemic proportions"

The risk factors for CAD are largely modifiable through the control of blood pressure, body weight, and blood levels of glucose and lipids. Of these, hypertension is a highly prevalent and important risk factor for CAD in the Western world, and recent clinical trials have reinforced our existing knowledge that prompt and effective blood pressure lowering, through drug treatment and lifestyle changes, can significantly reduce the risk of future cardiovascular disease and CAD. However, the influence of other risk factors in the pathogenesis of CAD must not be understated. Despite numerous attempts at prevention strategies, there has been no significant improvement in risk factor reduction for CAD. There is an urgent need for comprehensive screening, monitoring and treatment of the adult population, and for the implementation of programmes to promote more healthy ways of life. The education of doctors and patients alike in identifying and managing risk factors for CAD is vital if there is to be any lasting reduction in the prevalence of this disease.

"The risk factors for CAD are largely modifiable through the control of blood pressure, body weight, and blood levels of glucose and lipids"

There is a huge unmet clinical need in prevention and treatment of CAD, and greater collaboration between policy-makers, public health-surveillance and health-promotion organizations is required. The most immediate challenge, from a public health perspective, is to inform healthcare professionals and patients so that CAD risk factors can be sought, and risk reduction be optimized.

"Cardiovascular disease is largely preventable. We have the scientific knowledge to create a world in which most heart disease and stroke could be eliminated."

Victoria Declaration, arising from an Advisory Board of the International Heart Health Conference, 28th May 1992.

Lifestyle

> **Over half of population attributable risk of acute MI is due to lifestyle**

INTERHEART demonstrated that over half of population attributable risk of acute MI is due to lifestyle, specifically smoking, fruit and vegetable consumption, physical exercise and alcohol consumption.[18] The importance of a healthy, well-balanced diet combined with regular physical exercise, not smoking and moderation of alcohol consumption cannot be overemphasized. Reduction of these risk factors is often termed "primordial prevention" and should be addressed on a population-wide scale with national initiatives to improve diet, promote exercise and encourage smoking cessation. However, healthcare professionals should also encourage healthy lifestyle changes and provide support and encouragement as necessary.

Impact of lifestyle on cardiovascular risk factors

Diabetes

> **Diet and exercise are the cornerstones in the management of type 2 diabetes, and delaying its onset**

It has long been known that weight loss and physical activity can help improve blood sugar levels in individuals with diabetes. Recent evidence has shown that these interventions can also help to prevent or delay the onset of the disease. The benefits of such intervention, which were first demonstrated in the Chinese Da Qing study, have been confirmed in the Finnish Diabetes Prevention Study.[87,88] Both studies showed that an intensive lifestyle intervention consisting of weight loss and increased physical activity resulted in an identical 58% reduced risk of progressing from IGT to diabetes.

People at risk of developing diabetes and those who have established disease need to understand the importance of appropriate lifestyle, and that diet and exercise are the cornerstones in the management of type 2 diabetes, and delaying its onset (Figure 19).

Dyslipidaemia

> **Many patients with dyslipidaemia have concomitant obesity, particularly in those with diabetes**

Lifestyle interventions in patients with dyslipidaemia aim to reduce total and LDL-cholesterol concentrations, as well as providing an opportunity to address overall CAD risk factors, such as obesity and tobacco use. Many patients with dyslipidaemia have concomitant obesity, particularly in those with diabetes. Therefore, initial lifestyle measures include:
- weight reduction
- dietary reductions in saturated fat, simple sugars and alcohol
- increased physical activity.

Encouraging increased physical activity may help raise levels of protective HDL-cholesterol, which are characteristically low in patients with diabetes. Moderation of alcohol intake is especially important in patients who have high triglyceride levels.[89] More

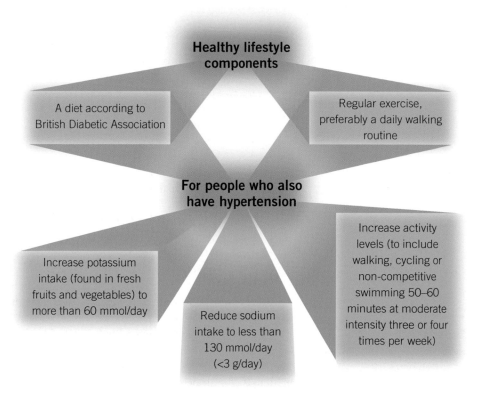

Healthy lifestyle components

A diet according to British Diabetic Association

Regular exercise, preferably a daily walking routine

For people who also have hypertension

Increase potassium intake (found in fresh fruits and vegetables) to more than 60 mmol/day

Reduce sodium intake to less than 130 mmol/day (<3 g/day)

Increase activity levels (to include walking, cycling or non-competitive swimming 50–60 minutes at moderate intensity three or four times per week)

intensive dietary interventions can be helpful in motivated patients and these patients benefit from the use of a multidisciplinary team including a dietitian (Figure 20).

Fig. 19 Lifestyle interventions that, if sustained, would lead to reduced cardiovascular risk, and minimize the need for drug therapy.

Hypertension

A number of contributing factors are recognized in hypertension. Alone these may be insufficient to account for development of hypertension, but are important because they may cause a further increase in blood pressure in certain patients, and can lessen the effectiveness of antihypertensive medication. Such factors include a high-salt diet, excess alcohol intake, obesity, physical inactivity and emotional stress. Measured programmes to enhance physical activity have been shown to cause significant and sustained blood pressure lowering. Elevated blood pressure is associated with insulin resistance, glucose intolerance and dyslipidaemia, such that Kaplan proposed a model to explain the interaction of what he called "the deadly quartet".[90] Although most patients with hypertension have multiple

31

Principle	Sources
Decrease total and saturated fat intake	Butter, hard margarine, whole milk, cream, ice cream, hard cheese, cream cheese, visible meat fat, usual cuts of red meat and pork, duck, goose, usual sausage, pastry, usual coffee whiteners, coconut, coconut oil, palm oil
Increase high-protein, low-saturated-fat foods	Fish, chicken, turkey, veal
Increase complex carbohydrates and fruit, vegetable and cereal fibre, with some emphasis on legumes	All fresh and frozen vegetables, all fresh fruit, all unrefined cereal foods, lentils, dried beans, rice
Moderately increase use of polyunsaturated and monounsaturated fats	Sunflower oil, corn oil, soya bean oil and products unless hardened (hydrogenated), olive oil
Decrease dietary cholesterol	Red meats, sweetbreads, kidneys, tongue, eggs (limit to 1–2 yolks per week), liver (limit to twice a month)
Moderately decrease sodium intake	Salt, sodium glutamate, cheese, tinned vegetables and meats, salt-preserved foods (ham, bacon, kippers), high-salt mineral waters, many convenience foods

Fig. 20 General principles of lipid-lowering diets.

Reproduced with permission from Galton D. Dyslipidaemia. Oxford: Elsevier, 2003. ©Elsevier

risk factors for CAD, the key step to minimizing their future risk is to control blood pressure to optimal target values.

A number of important lifestyle modifications are known to lower blood pressure, in addition to improving overall cardiovascular risk profile, as illustrated in Figure 21. Increased physical activity, weight loss, reduced dietary intake of salt and saturated fats, and increased dietary intake of fresh fruit and vegetables are capable of lowering blood pressure, albeit that the effect is modest in most patients. Moreover, these measures may delay the need to initiate drug therapy and, in patients already receiving drug therapy, are expected to enhance the efficacy of blood pressure lowering treatment.

High salt intake

There is a positive correlation between dietary salt intake and prevalence of hypertension across Western populations. In certain

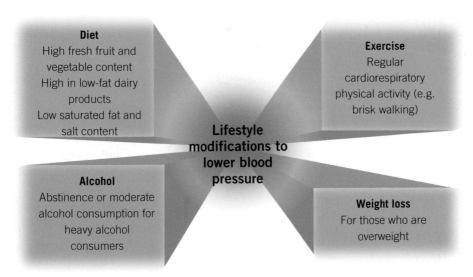

Diet
High fresh fruit and vegetable content
High in low-fat dairy products
Low saturated fat and salt content

Exercise
Regular cardiorespiratory physical activity (e.g. brisk walking)

Lifestyle modifications to lower blood pressure

Alcohol
Abstinence or moderate alcohol consumption for heavy alcohol consumers

Weight loss
For those who are overweight

patients, salt intake can have a significant impact on blood pressure, and this group are said to have "salt sensitive" hypertension. In this condition, a high versus low dietary intake of sodium salt can raise systolic blood pressure by 10 mmHg or more. Even in patients with hypertension who do not have salt sensitivity, excess dietary salt ingestion can exacerbate hypertension and diminish the effectiveness of certain treatments, particularly thiazide-type diuretics. Therefore, it is important to identify the possibility of excessive salt intake from the patient history. Strict salt restriction may cause a modest blood pressure lowering effect in some patients, and is likely to improve the blood pressure response to certain antihypertensive medications. Salt restriction alone is unlikely to cause a substantial blood pressure drop in any individual, but the consequent small blood pressure reduction is likely to significantly reduce the number of cardiovascular events in large populations. Furthermore, reduced salt intake may defer the need for pharmacotherapy in patients with borderline elevated blood pressure, or reduce the number of combination therapies required to control to target values in patients who are already established on treatment.

Fig. 21 Lifestyle modifications to lower blood pressure and enhance the efficacy of antihypertensive treatment.

66 Increased physical activity, weight loss, reduced dietary intake of salt and saturated fats, and increased dietary intake of fresh fruit and vegetables are capable of lowering blood pressure 99

Excess alcohol intake
Modest alcohol consumption appears generally safe, from a cardio-vascular risk perspective. However, heavy alcohol intake (more than three standard drinks per day) can play a significant role in the development of hypertension, particularly if excess consumption is

66 Heavy alcohol intake (more than three standard drinks per day) can play a significant role in the development of hypertension 99

sustained over a prolonged period. Ongoing alcohol excess worsens hypertension, antagonizes the effects of certain antihypertensive drugs, and further increases the risk of developing dilated cardiomyopathy. Substantial evidence demonstrates that reducing alcohol consumption is associated with a significant dose-dependent lowering of mean systolic and diastolic blood pressure, and that physician consultations provide an effective opportunity to reduce heavy drinking in hypertensive patients.[91] In patients who drink even more excessively, there is a heightened risk of non-compliance with antihypertensive and other medications. These findings highlight the importance of evaluating alcohol intake in new and existing patients with hypertension.

Dietary supplements
Omega-3 fatty acids
A number of randomized controlled trials have demonstrated that eating more oily fish or taking omega-3 polyunsaturated fatty acid supplementation improves survival in patients post MI.[92,93] A meta-analysis of 11 randomized controlled trials of 6–46 months' duration of omega-3 polyunsaturated fatty acid supplementation (nine trials) or increased fish intake (two trials) demonstrated significant reduction in all-cause mortality, fatal MI and sudden death, but not non-fatal MI.[94]

66 Eating more oily fish or taking omega-3 polyunsaturated fatty acid supplementation improves survival in patients post MI 99

Plant stanols
Plant stanols inhibit absorption of cholesterol from bile salt micelles in the small intestine and have been incorporated into a range of food stuffs such as margarine, yoghurt and milk. These products can provide a 10–15% reduction in LDL-cholesterol assuming 2–3 g are consumed per day providing a useful adjunct to medication or an alternative in those with only moderately raised LDL-cholesterol levels.

Bioactive dairy peptides
Dairy peptides such as Isoleucine-Proline-Proline (IPP) and Valine-Proline-Proline (VPP) have demonstrated some efficacy in reducing blood pressure. Dairy drinks containing these peptides have shown 7/4 mmHg reductions in blood pressure in patients with initially elevated levels, and as such can provide an option as part of a lifestyle regimen for patients with mildly elevated blood pressure (in the high normal range) to delay progression to hypertension.

66 Plant stanols inhibit absorption of cholesterol from bile salt micelles in the small intestine 99

Implementing lifestyle changes
Implementing lifestyle changes are real challenges to both the family physicians and patients.[95,96] Patients frequently require between five

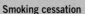

and ten attempts at changing a lifestyle before successfully learning how to change.[95,97] Failed attempts are therefore not a sign that future attempts will fail or are fruitless, but are a part of the change process.

Brief physician intervention approximately doubles the chances that a patient will incorporate some lifestyle changes.[95] Most lifestyle changes impact the whole family and involving the family in visits addressing lifestyle issues is advised. Involvement of a multidisciplinary team to provide support and reinforcement for the patient is also important.[98,99]

"Most lifestyle changes impact the whole family"

Conclusion

Lifestyle changes can be hard for many individuals to implement as bad habits are often ingrained. Support and advice from healthcare professionals can help to reinforce national healthy lifestyle initiatives and information on how adverse lifestyle choices are affecting individuals' health can encourage change. Details of how change can decrease an individual's risk of cardiovascular events and possibly prevent or delay the need for lifelong medication can also provide the necessary incentive.

"Support and advice from healthcare professionals can help to reinforce national healthy lifestyle initiatives"

Smoking cessation

Regular tobacco use has a major impact on overall cardiovascular risk, and is one of the key risk factors predisposing to CAD, aortic aneurysm, peripheral vascular disease and stroke. Cigarette smoke contains several thousand chemical constituents, many of which are implicated in causing tobacco-related disease. These include nicotine (an amine alkaloid compound), aromatic hydrocarbons, nitrosamines, vinyl chloride, formaldehyde, benzene and inorganic compounds, several of which can cause pro-mutagenic DNA changes or chromosomal abnormalities and are recognized potential carcinogens.[100,101] Cigarette smoke contains a large quantity of free radicals that promote oxidative stress, which can impair cardiovascular function and increase DNA susceptibility to mutation. The constituents of cigarette smoke mediate increased cardiovascular risk through a number of different mechanisms, such as enhanced platelet aggregability, altered haemoglobin oxygen-carrying capacity and impaired endothelium-dependent nitric oxide bioavailability.[102]

"Cigarette smoke contains several thousand chemical constituents"

Induction of a hypercoagulable state

Tobacco use affects both the coagulation cascade and platelet function. Inhalation of cigarette smoke leads to excess factor VII activity, which is responsible for initiation of coagulation and contributes to increased blood coagulability.[103] Furthermore, regular smokers have higher platelet thromboxane A_2 concentrations than non-smokers, which predisposes to increased platelet aggregability. Cigarette smoking is also associated with reduced platelet survival time, increased circulating platelet aggregates and release of platelet-specific proteins.[103] Plasma fibrinogen concentrations are typically higher in regular smokers; fibrinogen is a cofactor in platelet aggregation, and associated with increased blood viscosity.

> *Plasma fibrinogen concentrations are typically higher in regular smokers*

Reduced tissue oxygen delivery

Carbon monoxide is a combustion by-product that is inhaled during tobacco smoking. Regular cigarette smokers are said to have average carboxyhaemoglobin levels of about 5% per 20-pack smoked per day. These are significantly higher than the concentrations of 1–3% found in non-smokers as a result of exposure to everyday atmospheric pollution.[104] Carbon monoxide binds avidly to haemoglobin, thereby substantially reducing the oxygen-carrying capacity of circulating haemoglobin and compromising tissue oxygenation. In patients with established CAD exposure to carbon monoxide during exercise impairs ventricular function and predisposes to the development of arrhythmia.[105]

> *Exposure to carbon monoxide during exercise impairs ventricular function and predisposes to the development of arrhythmia*

Haemodynamic effects

Tobacco smoking causes constriction of the coronary arteries and increases total coronary vascular resistance, thereby exacerbating the inability of haemoglobin to carry oxygen efficiently. Rapid absorption of nicotine from cigarette smoke can produce immediate cardiovascular effects including increased heart rate and blood pressure, thereby increasing myocardial oxygen demand.[105]

Endothelial dysfunction

Cigarette smoking impairs endothelial function, which is thought to be an important early step in the initiation of atherosclerosis. Approximately 25% to 50% of the relation of cigarette smoking to the occurrence of CAD is attributable to the effect of smoking on fibrinogen concentrations in the blood.[106] High fibrinogen concentrations enhance the tendency for thrombosis, leading to occlusive clinical events. Smoking cessation results in decreased fibrinogen levels, reduced oxidative damage to the endothelium, and restored endothelial function.

> *Rapid absorption of nicotine from cigarette smoke can produce immediate cardiovascular effects*

Benefits of smoking cessation

Cessation of tobacco use restores several of the mechanisms that are characteristically impaired in regular tobacco users, including restoration of normal platelet aggregability and diminution of oxidative stress.[107,108]

Long-term cessation can offer substantial benefits in terms of cardiovascular risk. For example, in men aged <55 years, smoking abstinence for 1 year can reduce the risk of developing coronary heart disease by 50%, and risk is similar to non-smokers after as little as 2 years.[109] Smoking cessation decreases mortality from atherosclerotic disease by around 50% within 5 years in both men and women.[110] One study has found that overall mortality risk becomes similar to non-smokers after 10–14 years of persistent smoking abstinence.[111] However, among those who make unassisted attempts at smoking cessation, success rates are low and, for example, as few as 3–5% remain abstinent at 1 year.[112]

> *"Smoking cessation decreases mortality from atherosclerotic disease by around 50% within 5 years"*

Nicotine replacement therapy

Nicotine withdrawal and dependence are implicated in maintaining tobacco consumption and hindering attempts at quitting. Withdrawal symptoms are especially common among those who smoke every day or regularly smoke more than 10–15 cigarettes per day. Tobacco withdrawal symptoms include craving (61%), restlessness (46%), increased appetite or weight gain (45%) and irritability or anger (43%).[113] Nicotine replacement therapy can assist smoking cessation by replacing the nicotine formerly obtained from tobacco and is available in a number of preparations including gum, transdermal patches, nasal and sublingual sprays, and lozenges. The dose requirement depends on the usual nicotine consumption, which in turn depends on the amount of tobacco previously used. Generally, the initial dose is sufficiently high to suppress nicotine withdrawal symptoms, and then the dose is gradually reduced to zero as tobacco abstinence becomes established. Nicotine gum and lozenge preparations allow rapid absorption of nicotine, and can be used to counter acute cravings, whereas nicotine patches give a more sustained exposure over waking hours (patches are normally applied in the morning, and removed at bedtime). In the context of clinical trials, nicotine replacement therapy enhances the quit rate over and above that for unassisted attempts.

> *"Nicotine replacement therapy can assist smoking cessation by replacing the nicotine formerly obtained from tobacco"*

There has been concern about the possibility that nicotine replacement therapy might itself be cardiotoxic. It is important that the dose of treatment be kept to a minimum and used with particular caution in patients with established CAD. Of note, nicotine replacement therapy is currently contraindicated in women who are pregnant or breast-feeding.

> *"Nicotine replacement therapy enhances the quit rate over and above that for unassisted attempts"*

Bupropion

Bupropion is an atypical antidepressant that has been found to be effective in aiding smoking cessation. Currently it is the only non-nicotine treatment licensed to assist smoking cessation in the UK. Bupropion inhibits neuronal noradrenaline and dopamine uptake, and is thought to reduce tobacco withdrawal symptoms by enhancing central dopamine concentrations.[114] Bupropion treatment must be initiated 1–2 weeks before a planned smoking cessation date, and the intervening period should be used as an opportunity to offer motivational support. Two large randomized prospective studies found that bupropion increased 1-year quit rates from 12% on placebo to 23% on active treatment.[115,116]

> **" Bupropion treatment must be initiated 1–2 weeks before a planned smoking cessation date "**

Common adverse effects of bupropion include dry mouth, agitation, insomnia, headaches, dizziness and agitation. Seizures are a recognized feature, particularly if treated with higher than conventional doses.

Combined nicotine replacement therapy and bupropion

> **" Combination therapy might be helpful in certain patients "**

Both nicotine replacement therapy and bupropion appear equally effective as monotherapy. One study found that the combination of the two led to a higher quit rate at 1 year compared with either treatment alone.[116] The effectiveness of this strategy, and cost-effectiveness, are not yet established, but it appears as though combination therapy might be helpful in certain patients.

Obesity

Excess weight is a common risk factor for hypertension and diabetes, and is consequently important in the development of CAD and stroke. The increased prevalence of excess weight/obesity is predominantly due to changes in diet (increased fat and sugar intake) and an increasingly sedentary lifestyle. This is becoming a particular problem in children and young people. Excess weight can be reduced by healthy nutrition and regular physical exercise in most cases. Physical inactivity is linked to poor diet as a cause of obesity in many cases. The only way to increase food calories burned is to increase activity. However, many people at risk are unable to increase their activity level for a number of reasons:

> **" The only way to increase food calories burned is to increase activity "**

- osteoarthritis is highly prevalent in those over 65 years of age
- time demands and sedentary occupations
- fear of the unknown.

Many people are therefore unable to reverse their slide into metabolic imbalance and require drug therapy as part of their disease management.

There are a number of pathogenetic factors responsible for the development of hypertension in patients with obesity, including expansion of extracellular volume associated with relative and absolute

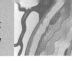

BMI = weight (kg) / height (m)^2
• Underweight <18.5 kg/m^2
• Normal 20–25 kg/m^2
• Overweight 25–30 kg/m^2
• Obese >30 kg/m^2

Fig. 22 Body mass index (BMI) cut-off points.

hypervolaemia and increased cardiac output, and activation of both the sympathetic nervous system and the renin-angiotensin-aldosterone system. It is suggested that obesity-related hypertension may be considered as a subset of essential hypertension and treated as a separate patient group. Of importance is the need to address obesity as an independent contributing risk factor in these patients, and a number of drug therapies are now available to assist weight loss. Orlistat and sibutramine have both been shown to be capable of aiding weight loss in highly selected obese patients. The use of orlistat in obese hypertensive patients is associated with a small decrease in blood pressure, whereas sibutramine may increase the blood pressure through effects on the central nervous system. There is little to choose between each drug in terms of weight loss alone and, therefore, orlistat is a preferred drug choice in obese patients with co-existent hypertension.[117]

> *A number of drug therapies are now available to assist weight loss*

Rimonabant is a selective cannabinoid-1 receptor (CB1) antagonist that has been shown to reduce body weight and improve the cardiovascular risk profile in obese patients. The RIO-Europe study in over 1500 patients with a body mass index (BMI) ≥30 kg/m^2 or BMI >27 kg/m^2 plus untreated dyslipidaemia, hypertension or both, demonstrated a significant increase in weight loss at 1 year with rimonabant 5 mg (-3.4 kg) or 20 mg (-6.6 kg) compared with placebo (-1.8 kg) all in addition to a hypocaloric diet.[118] The 20 mg dose also produced significant improvements in waist circumference, HDL-cholesterol, triglycerides and insulin resistance compared with placebo (Figure 23). The North-American arm of the RIO study recruited over 3000 patients with similar profiles to the European arm and found similar weight reductions with rimonabant (20 mg -6.3 kg vs -1.6 kg placebo) at the end of 1 year; however in patients switched from rimonabant to placebo in year 2 weight was regained suggesting that rimonabant should be taken continuously.[119] It should also be noted that there was a high drop-out rate limiting study of the longer-term effects of the drug.

> *Orlistat is a preferred drug choice in obese patients with co-existent hypertension*

There is also interest in the effects of rimonabant on smoking habits as it has been shown to double the odds of smoking cessation

Fig. 23 Change in HDL-cholesterol and triglycerides. One-year results of the RIO-Europe trial.[118] Reproduced with permission from Katz R, Purcell H. Acute Coronary Syndromes. Oxford: Elsevier, 2006. ©Elsevier

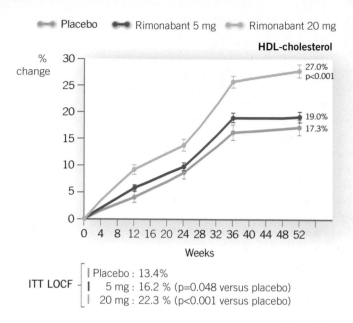

Placebo　　Rimonabant 5 mg　　Rimonabant 20 mg

ITT LOCF
Placebo : 13.4%
5 mg : 16.2 % (p=0.048 versus placebo)
20 mg : 22.3 % (p<0.001 versus placebo)

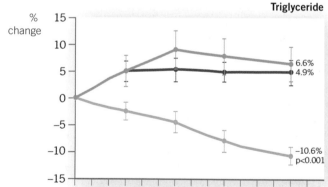

ITT LOCF
Placebo : 8.3 %
5 mg : 5.7 % (not significant versus placebo)
20 mg : −6.8 % (p<0.001 versus placebo)

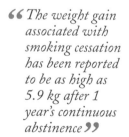

The weight gain associated with smoking cessation has been reported to be as high as 5.9 kg after 1 year's continuous abstinence

and reduce post-cessation weight gain.[120] As the weight gain associated with smoking cessation has been reported to be as high as 5.9 kg after 1 year's continuous abstinence and weight gain is reported as a common reason for relapse, rimonabant may provide a preferred option in some patients.

Diabetes mellitus
Epidemiology

Diabetes mellitus is one of the most prevalent diseases in the industrialized world, and the prevalence is rising in all populations. Around 5% of adults are known to have diabetes, which is likely to be a significant underestimation of true numbers with the disease. Worldwide, the number of patients with diabetes is expected to increase over the next decade, because of an ageing population and increased prevalence of obesity and sedentary lifestyles. Western lifestyle is moving away from what our physiology has evolved to cope with. As the lifestyle becomes "more feast than famine" and bouts of aerobic exercise become shorter and farther apart, muscle is lost and fat is gained, distorting normal physiology. People with greater expression of the "thrifty gene", may be better able to withstand a feast or famine existence.[121] However, when these people experience a "feast-always" existence, they are greatly predisposed to developing type 2 diabetes. Type 2 diabetes accounts for 90% of all cases of diabetes and is responsible for the increasing prevalence of diabetes we are seeing today.

There are many dire predictions about the coming onslaught on healthcare services from diabetes-fuelled morbidity combined with the ageing baby boom generation. These threats can be resolved to some extent by attention to risk factor modification and prevention. The coming "tsunami" of older people with diabetes will affect all of us in our everyday clinical practice, whether primary or specialty, and will also impact directly on healthcare budgets and the taxes we pay to support them. Diabetes, together with its related morbidity and associated death rates, has therefore been referred to as an epidemic. Not only is the prevalence of diabetes increasing, but the disease is occurring at younger ages, particularly in high-risk populations.[122] This leads to:

- more years at risk for developing the complications of diabetes
- complications developing at an earlier age and having an even more severe impact on the quality of life of those affected.

It has been estimated that the average person with diabetes has had the disease for 7–10 years before the diagnosis is made and about half of those diagnosed with diabetes already have a complication at the time of diagnosis.[123,124] The proportion of adults with diabetes mellitus is rising dramatically in the UK, Europe and worldwide, and is expected to do so well into this century (Figure 24).[125]

An important contributor to the increased prevalence of diabetes is the increasingly elderly population, and probably arises as a result of exposure to causal environmental and lifestyle factors for a longer period. This leads to a cumulative increase in the incidence of diabetes across progressively older members of society (Figure 25).[126]

"Western lifestyle is moving away from what our physiology has evolved to cope with"

"Type 2 diabetes accounts for 90% of all cases of diabetes"

"Not only is the prevalence of diabetes increasing, but the disease is occurring at younger ages"

41

Fig. 24 WHO data
indicating the
prevalence of diabetes
in 2000, and estimated
number of affected
patients in 2030.

Fig. 24 WHO data indicating the prevalence of diabetes in 2000, and estimated number of affected patients in 2030. Data from Ref 125.

	UK	Europe	World
Prevalence in 2000	1.8	33.3	171
Estimate for 2030	2.7	48.0	366
Percentage increase	**51%**	**44%**	**114%**

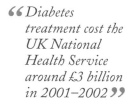

Fig. 25 Global diabetes prevalence by gender and age. Reproduced with permission from Wild S, Roglic G, Green A, et al. Global prevalence of diabetes: estimates for the year 2000 and projections for 2030. Diabetes Care 2004;27:1047–1053.

WHO data indicate that the excess global mortality attributable to diabetes in 2000 was about 2.9 million deaths, equivalent to 5.2% of all deaths in that year. Excess mortality attributable to diabetes accounted for 2–3% of deaths in the poorest countries and over 8% in the USA and other developed countries. In adults aged between 35 and 64 years, diabetes was responsible for between 6% and 27% of all deaths worldwide (Figure 26). In Europe, data from the year 2000 showed that diabetes mortality accounted for 9.5% of deaths in men aged 35–64 years, and 11.3% of deaths in women aged 35–64 years.[127] The relative mortality risk conferred by diabetes increases with progressively increasing age, which is in part due to increased prevalence in older populations (Figure 27).[127]

66 Diabetes treatment cost the UK National Health Service around £3 billion in 2001–2002 99

Financial burden of diabetes

In addition to the direct healthcare burden imposed by diabetes and its complications, there is a significant economic cost. Diabetes treatment cost the UK National Health Service (NHS) around £3 billion in 2001–2002, representing about 5% of all NHS spending. A significant proportion of this is used to provide healthcare for the complications of diabetes. For example, diabetes is responsible for over 30% of all

Relative mortality risk of diabetes			
	20–39 years	40–59 years	60–79 years
Women	5.5	3.5	2.5
Men	3.8	2.51	1.5

Fig. 26 The relative mortality risk of diabetes, compared with people without diabetes for men and women in different age groups in the UK in **2000.** Data from Ref 127.

—— Combined RR ━━ Lowest RR ━━ Highest RR

Number of deaths attributable to diabetes

1,200,000
1,000,000
800,000
600,000
400,000
200,000
0

0–19 20–29 30–39 40–49 50–59 60–69 70–79 80+

Age group (years)

Fig. 27 Variation in the number of deaths attributed to diabetes, according to lowest and highest relative mortality risks reported. RR = relative risk. Reproduced with permission from Roglic G, Unwin N, Bennett PH, et al. The burden of mortality attributable to diabetes: realistic estimates for the year 2000. Diabetes Care 2005;28:2130–2135.

prevalent cases of end-stage renal disease (ESRD).[128,129] This complication reduces the quantity and quality of patients' lives and places a heavy financial burden on healthcare systems.[130] The prevalence of diabetic nephropathy or transplantation in patients with diabetes is around 30% in the UK and 40% in the USA.[131] In the UK around 40% of all NHS expenditure on diabetes is directed toward treatment of diabetic nephropathy, which is estimated to be £765 million annually (range £657 million to £1.2 billion). In the UK annual healthcare costs associated with overt nephropathy were around £550 million in 2001–2002, and £190 million for end-stage renal failure. Comparable annual cost figures for the USA are approximately $9300 million and $3600 million for overt nephropathy and ESRD, respectively.[131]

A study in the Tayside region of Scotland found that patients with type 2 diabetes accounted for 6.6% of total prescriptions dispensed, representing 7.1% of the cost in the Tayside health region (5.5% excluding antidiabetic prescriptions).[132] There were higher proportionate drug costs in nearly all drug categories ranging from 2.6% higher (endocrine system) to 10.8% higher (cardiovascular), and

❝In the UK around 40% of all NHS expenditure on diabetes is directed toward treatment of diabetic nephropathy❞

patients with type 2 diabetes were 1.7 times more likely to be dispensed a drug item than those without diabetes. By extrapolation, the authors suggest that patients with diabetes account for approximately 8% of the UK drug budget, 90% of which is for those with type 2 diabetes. The relative risk of drug usage was even higher for patients with type 1 diabetes (2.1 times more likely to be dispensed a drug than those without diabetes).[132] However, given the lower prevalence of type 1 diabetes, the financial impact of treatment of patients with type 2 diabetes poses a substantially greater burden.

> *Most patients with diabetes or at risk of diabetes do not receive the best available therapies*

Despite knowledge about the pathophysiology of organ damage occurring in diabetes and the use of drugs and lifestyle changes to modify its course, most patients with diabetes or at risk of diabetes do not receive the best available therapies. Intensive medical treatment of patients with diabetes, particularly those with additional cardiovascular risk factors, significantly lowers the risk of end-stage microvascular and neuropathic conditions (by as much as 67–87%).[133] Dissemination of knowledge to patients and practitioners is now the immediate challenge for reducing diabetes-related morbidity and death.

Diabetes as a cardiovascular risk factor

Diabetes increases the risk of developing cardiovascular disease; for example type 2 diabetes is associated with a three- to fourfold increase

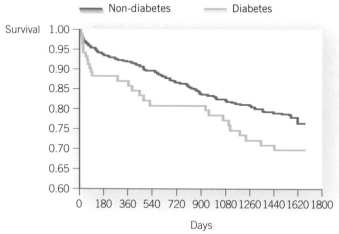

Fig. 28 Unadjusted Kaplan-Meier survival plots demonstrating significantly higher mortality rate in patients with diabetes compared to those without, from the PRAIS-UK study. Reproduced with permission from Bakhai A, Collinson J, Flather MD, et al. Diabetic patients with acute coronary syndromes in the UK: high risk and under treated. Results from the prospective registry of acute ischaemic syndromes in the UK (PRAIS-UK). Int J Cardiol 2005;100:79–84.

in CAD. It also has an adverse effect on outcome, as individuals with diabetes have a higher mortality rate from heart disease (Figure 28).[134] A number of large studies have shown unequivocally that diabetes mellitus confers a substantial increase in cardiovascular mortality and overall mortality:[135]

- two- to threefold increased cardiovascular risk in men
- three- to fivefold increased cardiovascular risk in women.

The independent effect of diabetes on incidence of acute MI or stroke is a 1.5- to twofold increase in men and a 1.5- to 6.5-fold increase in women.[136] In a cohort study from Scotland it was reported that, during a 7-year observation period, approximately 4% of patients with type 2 diabetes were admitted for acute MI.[137] In another study, patients with diabetes were found to have a 20–25% prevalence of acute MI during a follow-up of around 20 years.[136] The reason for the

Fig. 29 Major vascular complications associated with diabetes mellitus.
End-stage kidney disease, neuropathy and peripheral vascular disease photographs courtesy of Jonathan Bodansky. Diabetic retinopathy photograph courtesy of Graeme Catto, Izhar Khan and Paul Brown. Stroke photograph courtesy of Graham MacGregor and Michael Feher.

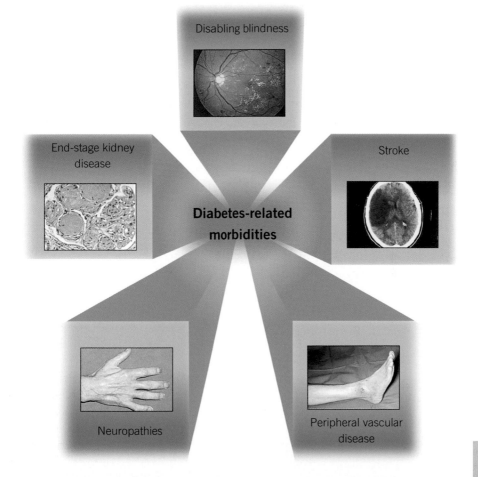

discrepancy is not clear. An analysis of the UK Prospective Diabetes Study (UKPDS) data reports that the adjusted rate of MI in persons with haemoglobin A_{1c} (HbA_{1c}) values between 9% and 10% is approximately twofold higher than that in people with normal HbA_{1c} concentrations.[138]

People with diabetes are exposed to increased risk of cardiovascular and renal disease (Figure 29). People with diabetes who also have other risk factors and markers of cardiovascular and renal disease have an even higher risk for cardiovascular events. The presence of these other risk factors also increases the likelihood of microvascular and macrovascular complications. Factors that adversely modify the long-term morbidity and mortality of people with diabetes are:

- high blood pressure
- abnormally high urine albumin levels including microalbuminuria

Fig. 30 Mechanisms thought to account for the vascular complications of diabetes.

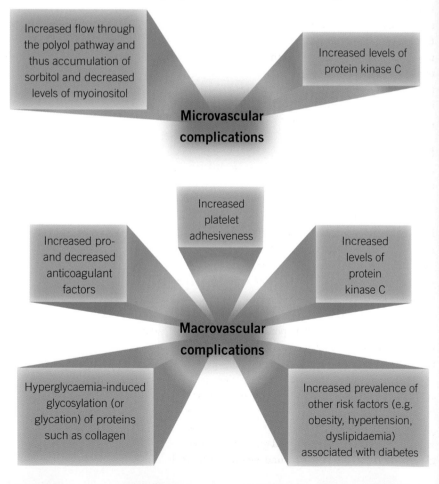

Increased flow through the polyol pathway and thus accumulation of sorbitol and decreased levels of myoinositol

Increased levels of protein kinase C

Microvascular complications

Increased platelet adhesiveness

Increased pro- and decreased anticoagulant factors

Increased levels of protein kinase C

Macrovascular complications

Hyperglycaemia-induced glycosylation (or glycation) of proteins such as collagen

Increased prevalence of other risk factors (e.g. obesity, hypertension, dyslipidaemia) associated with diabetes

- diabetic nephropathy
- abnormal blood lipids
- duration of diabetes
- lifestyle factors.

Some of the mechanisms thought to contribute to the development of microvascular and macrovascular complications of diabetes mellitus are outlined in Figure 30.

Clinical investigations in diabetes mellitus have historically focused on the glycaemic and metabolic consequences of the disorder. However, there is increasing recognition that diabetes mellitus is primarily a cardiovascular disorder with protean metabolic and atherogenic manifestations. Patients with diabetes are often found to have other cardiovascular risk factors present, including hypertension and dyslipidaemia, and this accelerates the progression of athero-sclerosis and its complications. For example, elevated blood pressure substantially increases CAD mortality in patients with diabetes, such that where both co-exist, there may be a 20–30% 10-year risk of a major cardiovascular event. Treatment of co-existent hypertension offers an opportunity to reduce mortality by as much as 34% in this patient group.[139–141] Given the large number of patients with diabetes in Western societies, the importance of early and effective blood pressure control to reduce CAD risk cannot be overstated.

❝Diabetes mellitus is primarily a cardiovascular disorder❞

❝Elevated blood pressure substantially increases CAD mortality in patients with diabetes❞

Early detection of diabetes by screening

At present only about half of all patients with diabetes are diagnosed before evidence of end-organ damage can be detected.[142] Given the strong familial predisposition for type 2 diabetes and the results of recent studies showing that diabetes can be prevented or delayed in high-risk individuals, it is important to identify patients at increased risk of developing diabetes.[143,144] This provides an opportunity for counselling on lifestyle modifications, and can allow early intervention to correct risk factors and prevent development of complications. Each physician has a role in helping to identify patients with, or at risk for, diabetes, its complications and co-morbid risk factors. The prevalence is rising much faster in certain populations, for example Aboriginal people, who appear to be at much higher risk, and screening programmes are especially important in such high-risk groups.[145,146]

As an example of effective screening, a prospective prevalence study was carried out in a urology outpatient clinic in a district general hospital serving a mixed urban and rural population.[147] Men presenting to the clinic with erectile dysfunction were recruited sequentially and underwent blood glucose measurements and dipstick glucose urinalysis screening for undiagnosed diabetes. In this

❝It is important to identify patients at increased risk of developing diabetes❞

47

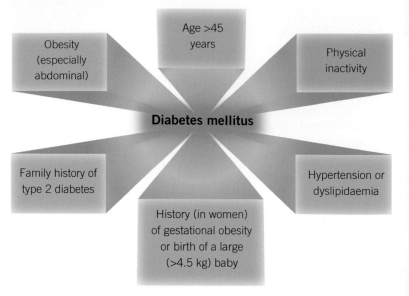

population the known diabetes prevalence was 17%. Among the remaining 107 men, 4.7% were found to have undiagnosed diabetes, and a further 12% were found to have IGT.[147] Therefore patients with erectile dysfunction were found to have a higher prevalence of undiagnosed diabetes than that expected in the general population. The study found that dipstick urinalysis, as a screening tool in this population, had sensitivity for diabetes of only 20%.

Assessing cardiovascular risk and prognosis

Routine screening for the presence of diabetes is recommended in those individuals at high risk. Known risk factors for the development of type 2 diabetes are listed in Figure 31.

Diabetes mellitus is a disease characterized by clustering of multiple cardiovascular risk factors. Consequently, therapeutic strategies to reduce CAD risk in patients with diabetes span a variety of different therapeutic areas that address:

- hyperglycaemia (control to target values)
- hypertension (treat to target blood pressures)
- microalbuminuria and nephropathy (detect and escalate therapy)
- dyslipidaemia (control to target values)
- erectile dysfunction (specific treatment may be needed).

A summary of treatment options for these conditions is presented in Figure 32, as used in the ongoing Diabetes Risk Assessment and Microalbuminuria (DREAM) 3 study.[148] In terms of cardiovascular risk factors, controlling hypertension and blood lipid levels in people

" Therapeutic strategies to reduce CAD risk in patients with diabetes span a variety of different therapeutic areas "

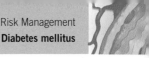

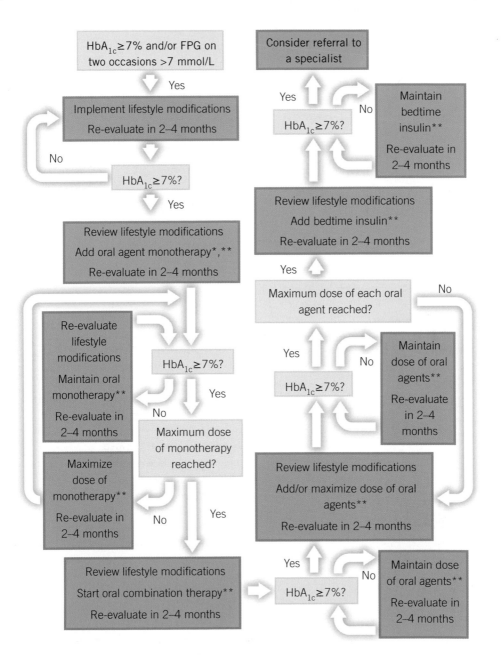

Fig. 32 Suggested management approach for glycaemic control, based on the protocol incorporated in the international DREAM study.[148] FPG = fasting plasma glucose. * Metformin is generally considered the preferred first-line agent. ** Symptomatic diabetic patients should be treated and/or referred to a specialist.

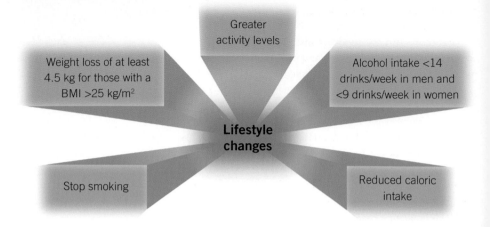

Fig. 33 Lifestyle intervention strategies aimed at improving insulin sensitivity, weight loss, blood pressure reduction, and lowering of overall cardiovascular risk.

with diabetes dramatically reduces the progression of vascular-related injury. This underpins the importance of adopting a multifactorial risk reduction approach for patients with diabetes.

Management: general principles

Ideally all patients with a new diagnosis of diabetes should be referred to an education centre for appropriate advice about the management of diabetes, including dietary intervention. A stepwise approach is advocated, with initial therapy consisting of lifestyle changes directed towards restoring insulin sensitivity and reducing overall cardiovascular risk (Figure 33). The individual with diabetes should receive adequate information and education so as to assume the key role in managing their illness with input from the primary care physician, diabetes nurse educator, dietitian, and diabetes and other specialists, with other professionals such as the podiatrist/chiropodist, being included in the team.

Recommendations should include strategies for improving adherence to prescribed medications. Self-monitoring of blood glucose is considered to be an integral component of diabetes management in patients requiring insulin but in patients receiving oral agents evidence for any benefits of self-monitoring is equivocal.[149] Self-monitoring of blood glucose cannot be considered as a stand-alone intervention; however, there is evidence that when used as part of a comprehensive educational strategy it can have an important role in improving metabolic control in patients receiving insulin.[150] Not only does it allow for appropriate titration of medication, it also provides important feedback to the person with diabetes on the immediate impact of lifestyle changes, promoting the individual's autonomy. Conversely in patients not treated with insulin, self-monitoring of blood glucose has

❝ The individual with diabetes should receive adequate information and education so as to assume the key role in managing their illness ❞

actually been shown to be associated with increased HbA_{1c} levels and psychosocial burden.

Self-monitoring needs to be considered within the context of a comprehensive self-care package and may not be appropriate for all patients. The frequency of testing should be individualized, but in general should be performed more frequently in the person receiving insulin or those taking oral agents associated with hypoglycaemia as a potential adverse effect. It is reasonable to expect that the regular feedback concerning medication dose titration and impact of lifestyle modifications provided by self-monitoring can improve adherence to medication and behaviour modification. It is also useful to remind patients of the additional benefits of monitoring their weight and diet, particularly with regard to blood pressure control and blood lipid levels.

With increasing time after diagnosis, some patients may become increasingly reliant upon antihyperglycaemic medications with less attention paid to maintaining healthy lifestyle measures. It is for this reason that refresher diabetes education sessions may be of value, and offer an opportunity to remind the patient of the varied potential benefits conferred by lifestyle intervention, for example blood pressure lowering, favourable effects on lipid profile and glycaemia, and general sense of well-being.

"Refresher diabetes education sessions may be of value, and offer an opportunity to remind the patient of the varied potential benefits conferred by lifestyle intervention"

Hyperglycaemia

Hyperglycaemia is thought to be an independent risk factor for progression of macrovascular complications including CAD and stroke, particularly in women. Hyperglycaemia is one of the hallmark metabolic abnormalities in diabetes and thought to underlie the development of:

"Hyperglycaemia is one of the hallmark metabolic abnormalities in diabetes"

- microvascular complications, which include retinopathy, nephropathy and neuropathy
- macrovascular complications, which include CAD, cerebrovascular disease and peripheral arterial disease.

Such is the importance of hyperglycaemia as an independent cardiovascular risk factor that Gerstein has recently used the term "dysglycaemia" to highlight the fact that blood glucose levels have a continuous and curvilinear relationship to cardiovascular risk, and that glucose concentrations even within the upper part of the normal reference range may be associated with increased risk.[151] A number of potential mechanisms are thought to be responsible for the vascular complications of hyperglycaemia, as illustrated in Figure 30.

"Blood glucose levels have a continuous and curvilinear relationship to cardiovascular risk"

Glycaemic control: pharmacological treatment

Because most of the increase in the prevalence of diabetes is of the type 2 variety, much of the related cardiovascular risk can be decreased

"Metformin is the generally preferred first-line agent"

"The microvascular complications of both type 1 and type 2 diabetes can be prevented to some extent by tight glycaemic control"

"Thiazolidinediones (glitazones) have also been shown to have similar (possibly greater) effects on cardiovascular risk markers to metformin"

by appropriate attention to risk factors. Management of patients who have diabetes includes treatment to optimize glucose and other risk factors, appropriate surveillance for target organ damage and referring appropriately when target organ damage is detected. Once diabetes is diagnosed, physicians should closely monitor:

- body weight
- blood pressure
- blood glucose
- blood lipids.

The control of blood glucose concentrations towards guideline targets involves implementation of lifestyle advice and, where necessary, introduction of one or more oral antihyperglycaemic agents and, if this is insufficient, the addition of, or replacement by, insulin therapy. If after a 4–8-week period of lifestyle change glucose levels are not in the optimal range, the addition of an oral hypoglycaemic agent should be considered (Figure 32). Metformin is the generally preferred first-line agent because its use in the UKPDS was associated with reduced cardiovascular complications in overweight patients.[152] If treatment goals are still not met, a second or even third oral agent can be added. If targets are still not met, bedtime insulin can be added. Finally if control is still suboptimal a switch to multiple doses of insulin should be made and sometimes an oral antihyperglycaemic agent added to an insulin-based regimen.

Research through peer review, industry–academia partnerships and industry-sponsored research is providing new evidence on an almost monthly basis to help us modify and improve treatments for diabetic patients. The microvascular complications of both type 1 and type 2 diabetes can be prevented to some extent by tight glycaemic control.[144,153] With regard to macrovascular disease, in the UKPDS the benefits of better blood pressure control outweighed those of improved glycaemic control, although it should be noted that the observed reductions in HbA_{1c} were relatively modest.

Evidence for benefit of insulin sensitizers on cardiovascular risk

It is thought that improving hyperglycaemia through insulin sensitivity provides enhanced cardiovascular protection compared with increasing insulin levels via direct insulin supplementation or increased insulin secretion. In the UKPDS trial metformin was the only diabetes medication associated with improved cardiovascular outcomes,[152] thought to be due to effects on fibrinolytic activity secondary to either improved insulin sensitivity or lower insulin concentrations. Thiazolidinediones, such as pioglitazone and rosiglitazone (glitazones), have also been shown to have similar (possibly greater)

effects on cardiovascular risk markers to metformin leading to postulation that they may also provide cardiovascular benefit.[41] However, this has yet to be conclusively proven in a large randomized controlled trial.

Pioglitazone has been shown to significantly reduce diastolic blood pressure (p=0.016) compared with placebo in 60 non-diabetic patients with arterial hypertension.[154] Improvements in the lipid profile were also observed. Furthermore the PIONEER study, which compared pioglitazone and glimepiride, suggests that the reduction in cardiovascular risk markers, such as LDL/HDL ratio, high-sensitivity CRP (hsCRP) and carotid intima-media thickness seen in type 2 diabetes patients is independent of improvement in glycaemic control.[155]

The PROactive study investigated the effect of adding either pioglitazone or placebo to existing medication on macrovascular complications of type 2 diabetes.[156] While an improvement in the primary outcome – a composite of all-cause mortality, non-fatal MI (including silent MI), stroke, acute coronary syndrome, endovascular or surgical intervention in the coronary or leg arteries, and amputation above the ankle – was observed, it failed to reach statistical significance (hazard ratio [HR] 0.90, 95% CI 0.80–1.02, p=0.095). However the secondary endpoint – a composite of all-cause mortality, non-fatal MI and stroke – did demonstrate a significant improvement in favour of pioglitazone (HR 0.84, 95% CI 0.72–0.98, p=0.027), although the importance of this is unclear due to the absence of significance in the primary endpoint.[157]

Rosiglitazone has been shown to improve postprandial triglyceride and free fatty acid metabolism in people with type 2 diabetes,[158] but not to reduce overall triglyceride levels. Rosiglitazone has also demonstrated significant reduction in both systolic and diastolic blood pressure in non-diabetic hypertensive patients as well as favourable changes in other cardiovascular risk markers.[159] However a comparison of rosiglitazone and pioglitazone in combination with glimepiride in patients with type 2 diabetes and metabolic syndrome found that pioglitazone, but not rosiglitazone, significantly improved lipid and lipoprotein variables,[160] suggesting that the two drugs may have different effects on cardiovascular risk.

Trials assessing the effect of rosiglitazone on cardiovascular outcomes are currently in progress. The RECORD study is a 6-year, randomized open-label study in type 2 diabetes patients that should provide robust data on the extent to which rosiglitazone, in combination with metformin or sulphonylurea therapy, affects cardiovascular outcomes.[161] In addition the GATE study should establish any benefit of rosiglitazone on endothelial function.[162]

> *Pioglitazone has been shown to significantly reduce diastolic blood pressure compared with placebo* "

> *Rosiglitazone has been shown to improve postprandial triglyceride and free fatty acid metabolism* "

> *Interest in the PPAR group of receptors has increased and dual PPAR alpha and gamma agonists have been developed* "

53

Future antihyperglycaemic agents

Following the success of glitazones (peroxisome proliferators-activated receptor (PPAR) gamma agonists) and fibrates (PPAR alpha agonists), interest in the PPAR group of receptors has increased and dual PPAR alpha and gamma agonists have been developed, known as "glitazars". These compounds appear to have beneficial effects on laboratory values for both insulin sensitivity and lipid profiles, suggesting the potential to provide greater cardiovascular benefit than the glitazones. However concerns have been raised regarding a possible adverse effect on cardiovascular mortality with one agent, muraglitazar,[163] resulting in the US Food and Drug Administration (FDA) requesting more long-term data on cardiovascular outcomes. It is not currently clear whether these concerns are class related or specific to muraglitazar; however they are likely to also result in delays to the approval of other products, such as tesaglitazar.

Other novel agents in development for the treatment of diabetes include glucagon-like protein-1 (GLP-1) receptor agonists and dipeptidyl peptidase IV (DPP IV) antagonists. GLP-1 agonism can also reduce food intake and trials of the injectable GLP-1 analogue exenatide have demonstrated improved glycaemic control without inducing weight gain in those previously uncontrolled with oral therapy.[164] Indeed exenatide has actually been shown to promote weight loss providing the potential to improve cardiovascular risk factors.[165] DPP IV inhibitors are available in oral formulations and, as well as lowering glucose levels, have shown potential in preventing or delaying the development of overt diabetes in those at risk.[165]

Glycaemic control: therapeutic targets

Increasing epidemiological data and clinical trial evidence show that tight glucose control delays the progression of microvascular and macrovascular complications of diabetes. Current recommendations for glycaemic targets define optimal glycaemic control as HbA_{1c} <6.5%.[166]

The optimal HbA_{1c} target of <6.5%, rather than "normal" HbA_{1c} levels, recognizes that it is often difficult to achieve "normal" levels without incurring a serious risk of intermittent hypoglycaemia, especially in patients with type 1 diabetes. An epidemiological analysis of the UKPDS found no minimum HbA_{1c} value beyond which there were no further benefits from glucose lowering.[152] Therefore it appears that any reduction in HbA_{1c} might be associated with a reduced risk of both microvascular and macrovascular complications. In their analysis every 1% decrease in HbA_{1c} was associated with a 25% reduction in risk for MI.[152] Although HbA_{1c} is considered to be the best measure of overall glycaemic control, blood or capillary glucose levels are still

> **❝Exenatide has been shown to promote weight loss providing the potential to improve cardiovascular risk factors❞**

> **❝DPP IV inhibitors have shown potential in preventing or delaying the development of overt diabetes in those at risk❞**

> **❝Any reduction in HbA_{1c} might be associated with a reduced risk of both microvascular and macrovascular complications❞**

important to safely and effectively manage the doses of oral hypo-glycaemic agents and insulin. Useful information can be gained by studying blood glucose measurements obtained by patient self-monitoring at various times of day.

Microalbuminuria

Microalbuminuria is a marker of glomerular damage, which is now considered to be the earliest detectable stage of kidney disease in diabetes.[167] Urine albumin, which escapes the glomerulus, is a mediator as well as a marker of further renal damage. Over time urine albumin excretion increases. When the daily urine albumin excretion is greater than >300 mg/day (200 mg/L) the patient is said to have overt diabetic nephropathy. Abnormally high urine albumin in those with and without diabetes is a powerful prognostic factor for long-term mortality rates.[168] The risk of ESRD is nine times higher in people with diabetes, even when other risk factors such as blood pressure and lipid levels are controlled.[169]

Microalbuminuria indicates a higher risk of cardiovascular events as well as an increased risk of developing diabetic nephropathy. In a review by Eastman and Keen microalbuminuria was associated with a 10-fold increased risk of cardiovascular events, making it a more powerful marker than hypertension, elevated cholesterol or smoking.[170] Microalbuminuria has been shown to be the leading predictor of coronary heart disease mortality rates in patients with type 2 diabetes.[170] This does not imply that microalbuminuria is a mediator, but rather a marker of cardiovascular risk. Damsgaard *et al* also demonstrated that microalbuminuria is a marker of cardiovascular risk. In a cohort of elderly people with type 2 diabetes followed for over 8 years, microalbuminuria was a strong predictor of coronary events.[168] Interestingly, higher cardiovascular risk has also been shown in non-diabetic people with microalbuminuria.[171]

Diagnosis

Microalbuminuria develops in 20–30% of patients with type 2 diabetes.[172,173] Normally urine albumin excretion is <30 mg/day. Standard urine dipsticks become positive for albumin when the daily urine excretion exceeds 300 mg/day. When this occurs in patients with diabetes it signifies diabetic nephropathy, macroalbuminuria or overt nephropathy.[174,175] Individuals who have urinary albumin excretion rates that lie between normal albuminuria and diabetic nephropathy are said to have microalbuminuria (30–300 mg/day). Because the standard urine dipsticks normally do not detect such low levels of urine albumin, measurement of urine in the microalbuminuria range (Figure

> *Microalbuminuria is now considered to be the earliest detectable stage of kidney disease in diabetes*

> *Higher cardiovascular risk has also been shown in non-diabetic people with micro-albuminuria*

> *Measurement of urine in the microalbuminuria range requires laboratory analysis*

55

Definition	Urine albumin by dipstick (protein)	Spot urine (mg/L)	Screening test (albumin/creatinine ratio) (mg/µmol)		Confirmation test	
			Men	Women	24-h urine (mg/24h)	Night collection (mg/min)
Normal	Negative	<20	<2.0	<2.8	10+3	7+2
Normoalbuminuria	Negative	<20	<2.0	<2.8	<30	<20
Microalbuminuria	Negative	20–200	2.0–20	2.8–28	30–300	20–200
Macroalbuminuria	Positive	>200	>20	>28	>300	>200

Fig. 34 Categories of urinary albumin excretion, as determined by dipstick urinalysis, isolated urine sample analyses, or prolonged urine collection.

34) requires laboratory analysis.[175] Repeat spot urine tests for albumin to creatinine ratios (>2–3 is abnormal) are sensitive for the diagnosis of microalbuminuria (Figure 35).[176]

Microalbuminuria and cardiovascular risk

Fig. 35 Methods for detection of microalbuminuria and overt diabetic nephropathy.

The threshold for initiating treatment for microalbuminuria is a urine albumin level of 30 mg/day or 20 mg/L independent of blood pressure. Urine albumin levels should be monitored regularly in all people with diabetes. Monitoring should begin immediately in all patients with type 2 diabetes, and 5 years after the diagnosis is established in patients with type 1 diabetes. A series of clinical practice guidelines now call for screening for microalbuminuria so that patients at risk can be identified and started on therapy.[177–180] Levels of urine albumin are, of course, a continuum from 0 to the nephrotic range, but this continuum is broken down into artificial groupings based on the results of clinical

Category	24-hour albumin (mg)	Albumin concentration (mg/L)	Albumin/creatinine (mg/mol) – men/women
Normal	<30	<20	<2.0/<2.8
Microalbuminuria	30–300	20–200	2.0–20/2.8–28
Overt nephropathy	>300	>200	>20/>28

observations.[181] Higher concentrations of urine albumin within each category indicate a worse renal and cardiovascular prognosis.[182,183] For example patients with diabetes who have urine albumin concentrations of 20–30 mg/day are more likely to progress to microalbuminuria than those with excretion of <10 mg/day, although both groups fall within the normal range for albumin excretion rates <30 mg/day.[184] When microalbuminuria is present, high systolic blood pressure appears to play an important role in accelerating the progression to overt diabetic nephropathy.[185]

Management of microalbuminuria
A treatment algorithm for microalbuminuria is presented in Figure 36, based on the ongoing DREAM study protocol.[148] Microalbuminuria is now an indication for initiating an angiotensin-converting enzyme (ACE) inhibitor, even in the presence of "normal" blood pressure.

> *Microalbuminuria is now an indication for initiating an ACE inhibitor, even in the presence of 'normal' blood pressure*

Target values
The goal of therapy for microalbuminuria is to reduce the urine albumin excretion rate by 50% or more; such a reduction has been associated with a lower rate of deterioration of renal function.[186] The goal of treatment in diabetic patients with microalbuminuria is to reduce cardiovascular–renal risk through multiple risk factor reduction. In patients whose blood pressures have been brought towards or to target and who are on an ACE inhibitor, a fall in urine albumin excretion of 50% is a good prognostic marker.[187]

> *Once a patient has been started on therapy, the assessment of effects on urinary albumin excretion may be helpful but is secondary to attaining good blood pressure control*

Pharmacological therapies
There is now evidence that anti-angiotensin II therapy with ACE inhibitors can delay progression of microalbuminuria to diabetic nephropathy and even cause regression of urine albumin excretion to normal levels again. Patients with diabetes and microalbuminuria should be treated with an ACE inhibitor or an angiotensin II receptor antagonist (AIIRA). Once a patient has been started on therapy, the assessment of effects on urinary albumin excretion may be helpful but is secondary to attaining good blood pressure control.

Primary prevention of microalbuminuria
In type 1 diabetes progression to microalbuminuria can be delayed or prevented by attaining good glycaemic control and utilizing an ACE inhibitor.[144,188] In type 2 diabetes, progression to microalbuminuria may be delayed more effectively by adequate blood pressure control than by controlling blood glucose alone.[138] ACE inhibition delays progression from normal albumin excretion to microalbuminuria.[189]

> *ACE inhibition delays progression from normal albumin excretion to micro-albuminuria*

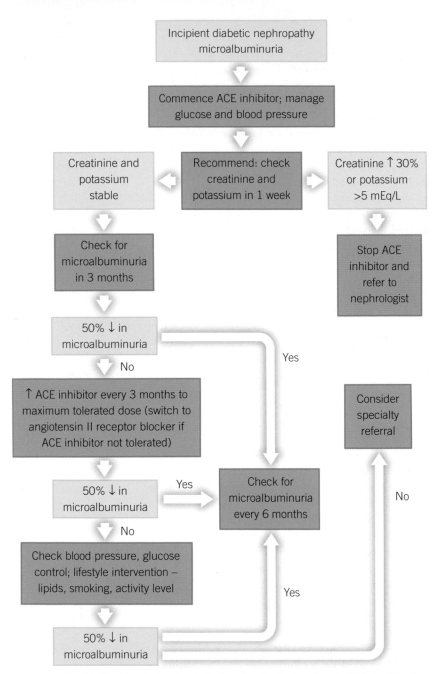

Fig. 36 Algorithm for treatment of microalbuminuria, based on the Diabetes Risk Assessment and Microalbuminuria (DREAM) study.[148]

Preventing progression from microalbuminuria to diabetic nephropathy

In type 1 diabetes a number of well-conducted placebo-controlled trials have demonstrated the effectiveness of ACE inhibition in preventing progression to diabetic nephropathy.[190] In patients with type 2 diabetes and normal blood pressure ACE inhibitors reduced the risk of progression from microalbuminuria to diabetic nephropathy by around 30% over 5 years, which was confirmed in another small study.[191,192] Until recently only small studies had reported on treatments to delay progression to nephropathy in patients with type 2 diabetes with hypertension.[193–197] In the HOPE study ACE inhibitors reduced the absolute risk of progression to diabetic nephropathy by 1.9% over 4.5 years.[189] In a controlled trial of 590 hypertensive patients with type 2 diabetes, the IRMA II study showed that AIIRA therapy delayed the decline in renal function in this high-risk group.[198] Irbesartan reduced the risk of progression from microalbuminuria to diabetic nephropathy by around 50%, an effect that was independent of any change in blood pressure. The findings were consistent with those expected from earlier trials with ACE inhibitors, suggesting that either class of drugs is equally effective.[199] In type 2 diabetes there have been no clinical trials in which ACE inhibitors and AIIRA therapy have been compared directly, or studied in combination. The ONTARGET study underway in early 2002 will address this issue as a secondary question.[200]

“In type 2 diabetes there have been no clinical trials in which ACE inhibitors and AIIRA therapy have been compared directly, or studied in combination”

Monitoring pharmacological therapy of microalbuminuria

Urine albumin excretion levels are a cardiovascular risk marker, and highlight the need to address major cardiovascular risk factors (i.e. blood pressure, serum lipids, blood sugar, ongoing tobacco use). Initially it might be reasonable to test every 3 months and if urine albumin excretion rate is still excessive then the adequacy of therapy for established cardiovascular risk factors should be reviewed and intensified. Once therapy for these risk factors is established and microalbuminuria persists then it is reasonable to increase the dose of ACE inhibitor or AIIRA therapy towards the maximum recommended dosages, and the combination of the two might be helpful in certain situations. Once therapy has been optimized urine albumin can be assessed annually as a means of monitoring progression to overt diabetic nephropathy.

“Once therapy has been optimized urine albumin can be assessed annually”

Combination therapy in microalbuminuria

When comparing ACE inhibitors and AIIRAs to other blood pressure lowering agents there is evidence for their superiority for delaying progression of nephropathy. However, in most cases multiple drug combinations will be required to attain adequate blood pressure

“The combination of a calcium-channel blocker and ACE inhibitor appears effective in reducing cardiovascular risk compared with either agent alone”

control.[180,201] The combination of a calcium-channel blocker and ACE inhibitor appears effective in reducing cardiovascular risk compared with either agent alone, and the combination appears beneficial in reducing urine albumin excretion.[202–207]

> ❝ *It is unclear if dual blockade of the renin-angiotensin-aldosterone system has an effect independent of blood pressure lowering alone* ❞

A pragmatic summary of the existing evidence is:
- to use ACE inhibitors in patients with diabetes and microalbuminuria, whether hypertensive or not
- to use AIIRA if ACE inhibitor is not tolerated
- AIIRAs have accumulated a greater body of evidence to support their role in patients with co-existent hypertension and left ventricular hypertrophy, and might be a preferred alternative in these patients.

There may be additional benefits from combining the two classes, particularly if urine albumin excretion has not fallen, but it is unclear if dual blockade of the renin-angiotensin-aldosterone system has an effect independent of blood pressure lowering alone.[208] The apparent benefit of combining the two agents might reflect inadequate doses of each agent alone. Escalation beyond conventional doses might be appropriate in this patient group, especially if the renoprotective effects are truly independent of blood pressure mechanisms, but this requires further evaluation.

Diabetic nephropathy

Importance of diabetic nephropathy as a cardiovascular risk factor

The finding of diabetic nephropathy indicates a very high risk of progression to ESRD. It also indicates a high likelihood of cardiovascular events, which places patients at similar risk as those who have had a previous MI.[26]

> ❝ *Massive disruption of the size and barrier functions of the glomerulus allows increasingly larger quantities of albumin to spill into the urine* ❞

Epidemiology and pathophysiology

Of diabetic patients with microalbuminuria, 50% will develop diabetic nephropathy within 10 years of diagnosis.[209–212] In the Micro-HOPE study the risk of developing diabetic nephropathy over the course of the study (5 years) was 20% for those with microalbuminuria and 2% for those without. These rates are essentially the same for both type 1 and type 2 diabetes.[213–218]

Hyperglycaemia-induced sclerosis of the afferent arteriole results in haemodynamic changes that cause elevated glomerular capillary pressure. The combination of raised intraglomerular pressure and diabetes-mediated glomerular mesangial cell alterations result in focal glomerulosclerosis, and the appearance of Kimmelstiel–Wilson lesions, which are pathognomonic of diabetic nephropathy (Figure 37).

Massive disruption of the size and barrier functions of the glomerulus allows increasingly larger quantities of albumin to spill into

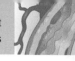

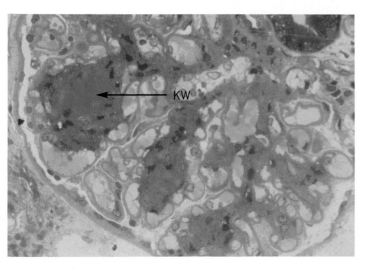

Fig. 37 Light microscopy of renal biopsy material from a patient with type 2 diabetes and hypertension. The arrow indicates focal segmental glomerulosclerosis, so-called Kimmelstiel–Wilson lesion. Photo courtesy of the Wellcome Trust.

the urine. Eventually the most severely affected glomeruli become obsolete. The remaining nephrons increase their single nephron glomerular filtration rate, which partially accommodates the loss of nephron numbers. However as the surviving nephrons increase their glomerular capillary pressures the process is accelerated.

The accumulated renal damage leads to hypertension, in part through sodium retention and activation of the renin-angiotensin-aldosterone cascade, and via other mechanisms that remain unclear. High blood pressure leads to even higher intraglomerular pressures, transmitted by the sclerosed afferent arterioles, promoting further renal injury and setting up a positive feedback loop causing an inexorable decline in renal function. Patients who develop diabetic nephropathy will eventually develop ESRD, if they do not die of other causes.[213] ESRD occurs in around 20% of patients with type 1 diabetes after 30 years of disease, while those with type 2 diabetes have a lifetime risk of around 10%.[219–221]

Urine albumin excretion reflects an increasing continuum of risk of both kidney and cardiovascular disease. Mortality rates in patients with diabetic nephropathy are significantly higher than in patients with microalbuminuria. Untreated, the decline in glomerular filtration rate in patients with diabetic nephropathy is around 10 mL/min per year.[222] So, for example if a patient has baseline glomerular filtration rate of 100 mL/min, then renal replacement therapy can be anticipated within 10 years. Control of blood pressure, treating microalbuminuria and targeting other cardiovascular risk factors are likely to reduce this rate of decline.[222]

66Patients who develop diabetic nephropathy will eventually develop ESRD, if they do not die of other causes 99

61

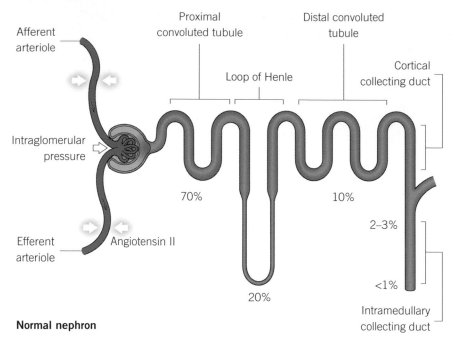

Afferent arteriole

Proximal convoluted tubule

Distal convoluted tubule

Cortical collecting duct

Loop of Henle

Intraglomerular pressure

70%

10%

2–3%

Efferent arteriole

Angiotensin II

20%

<1%

Intramedullary collecting duct

Normal nephron

Fig. 38a Schematic showing normal nephron.

Management of diabetic nephropathy

When diabetic nephropathy becomes established it is thought that intervention can hope to delay progression, rather than correct normal function. If patients are identified early enough the time of progression to ESRD can be dramatically delayed. Even in patients with very advanced diabetic nephropathy the time to ESRD may be doubled by the use of appropriate treatment. Given that a median survival rate of elderly patients (>65 years old) with diabetes and ESRD is only 2 years, any delay in the progression to ESRD can have a substantial impact.[223]

❝ Intervention can hope to delay progression, rather than correct normal function ❞

Target values

A key goal in reducing the progression of diabetic nephropathy is to attain strict blood pressure target values (<130/80 mmHg), and to institute multiple risk factor interventions including smoking cessation, cholesterol lowering and glycaemic control.

Non-pharmacological therapies

The advice of a dietitian should be provided for patients with established diabetic nephropathy. In addition to drug therapy, general

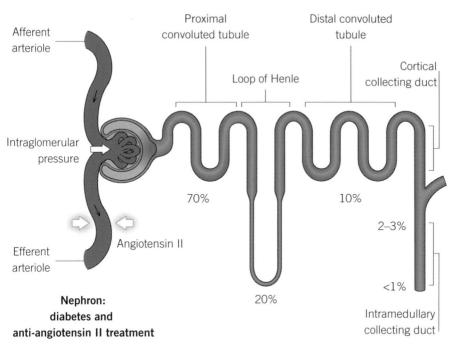

Fig. 38b The nephron in a patient with type 2 diabetes. ACE inhibitor and AIIRA therapy block the effects of angiotensin II on the efferent arteriole and thereby reduce glomerular pressure (excess glomerular pressure is thought to contribute to development of diabetic nephropathy). Note that this mechanism is protective in situations where there is excess afferent arteriolar pressure, but potentially deleterious in situations where there is inadequate arteriolar pressure (for example renal artery stenosis).

advice for patients with diabetic nephropathy is to avoid a high protein diet because this might cause further dilatation in the afferent arteriole and accelerate renal dysfunction.[224]

Pharmacological therapies

Treatment of diabetic nephropathy starts with an ACE inhibitor or AIIRA in patients with type 2 diabetes, irrespective of baseline blood pressure. This blocks angiotensin II-mediated vasoconstriction of the efferent arteriole, thereby decompressing the glomerulus and reducing the risk of haemodynamic damage (Figure 38). In addition therapy might restore renal function through other mechanisms, for example direct humoral effects of angiotensin II blockade on mesangial cell function.

66Therapy might restore renal function through other mechanisms 99

The largest clinical trial in type 1 diabetic nephropathy found that ACE inhibitor treatment caused a 50% reduction in a composite endpoint of death, dialysis and doubling of the creatinine level. This benefit was thought to be independent of blood pressure lowering.[225] The IDNT and RENAAL trials included patients with hypertension, type 2 diabetes and established diabetic nephropathy, and studied the effects of irbesartan and losartan, respectively, versus an active comparator (amlodipine and atenolol, respectively). Together, these studies recruited over 3200 patients for a minimum of 2 years, and showed that AIIRA therapy reduced a composite endpoint including death, dialysis and doubling of creatinine level. These effects could not be explained by changes in blood pressure.

Combination therapy

The difficulty in controlling blood pressure in advanced diabetic nephropathy was illustrated in the IDNT and RENAAL studies. In both trials, an average of three medications was required to control blood pressure to target. Therefore in order to attain blood pressure targets of <130/80 mmHg in patients with diabetes, combination therapy is required in the majority.

In Micro-HOPE, a substudy of the HOPE trial, 3577 people with diabetes who had had previous cardiovascular events or had one major cardiovascular risk factor were randomly assigned to the ACE inhibitor ramipril or placebo.[189] After 4.5 years of follow-up there was a 24% risk reduction of overt nephropathy. A meta-analysis of previous ACE inhibitor studies gave similar results.[140]

Assuming that an ACE inhibitor or AIIRA has been started as initial therapy, what is the next step? Given the blood pressure-lowering synergy of ACE inhibitors and AIIRAs with diuretics, addition of a low-dose thiazide (for example hydrochlorothiazide 12.5–25 mg/day or bendroflumethiazide 2.5 mg daily), or a long-acting calcium channel blocker (for example long-acting nifedipine 30 mg daily or amlodipine 10 mg daily). Although some studies have found urine albumin excretion increased when a calcium channel blocker was used as monotherapy, this occurred only in patients with poorly controlled blood pressure.[226] Earlier studies had suggested that calcium channel blocker monotherapy might increase cardiovascular event rates, in patients with and without diabetes, perhaps through excess heart failure.[227–230] However there is also a high level of evidence indicating that calcium channel blockers reduce mortality rates in patients with diabetes and ISH.[203] An analysis of patients with diabetes in the HOT study who received a long-acting calcium channel blocker as the first drug as part of a "stepped protocol" approach found a reduction of cardiovascular events with lower blood pressure.[202] In the IDNT study the amlodipine arm performed as well as the AIIRA and control arms for cardiovascular events and overall

> **In order to attain blood pressure targets of <130/80 mmHg in patients with diabetes, combination therapy is required in the majority**

> **There is also a high level of evidence indicating that calcium channel blockers reduce mortality rates in patients with diabetes and ISH**

mortality rate, and demonstrated a greater reduction in the incidence of MI when compared with the irbesartan arm.[231] Most of the controversy surrounding the use of calcium channel blockers in patients with diabetes is based on trials in which these agents are used as monotherapy, and current data suggest that addition of a long-acting dihydropyridine calcium channel blocker to an ACE inhibitor or AIIRA provides an effective means of blood pressure lowering and cardiovascular risk reduction. In FACET, of the patients who received both an ACE inhibitor and amlodipine in combination, around one third showed a trend towards better outcomes than patients who received either agent alone.[227]

Need for specialist intervention

It is important for the primary care physician to arrange for appropriate surveillance of patients for the development of disease complications. Such patients must be referred for appropriate specialist management when target organ damage is detected. Routine referral for detailed retinal examination on an annual basis, and to a foot clinic for regular examination of the feet are means of detecting complications early and also cost-effective. The practitioner must be on the constant lookout for evidence of macrovascular complications of diabetes. For example, angina might be present and associated with less prominent symptoms than typically reported by patients free of diabetes. Symptoms and signs of peripheral vascular disease should be sought to enable early detection and treatment, so as to avoid unnecessary amputations associated with late disease manifestation.

It is wise to refer patients to the local nephrologist when their renal function has begun to deteriorate (i.e. glomerular filtration rate <60 mL/min or creatinine >130 mmol/L). By providing additional patient information, the multidisciplinary teams associated with most nephrology units have been demonstrated to delay the onset of ESRD by as much as 6 months.[232] It seems reasonable to refer patients to a blood pressure specialist for review if blood pressure control has not been achieved with three antihypertensive drugs in combination.

Summary

Diabetes increases the risk of developing cardiovascular disease. Diabetes and hypertension are often associated and together can lead to CAD, stroke, peripheral vascular disease, nephropathy and retinopathy. Hypertension incidence increases by 3% for each year of diabetes, and is three times more likely in patients with proteinuria and 23% more likely in those with higher HbA_{1c} levels.[233] Clinical trials have shown that blood pressure control to target values, good

"Current data suggest that addition of a long-acting dihydropyridine calcium channel blocker to an ACE inhibitor or AIIRA provides an effective means of blood pressure lowering and cardiovascular risk reduction"

"The practitioner must be on the constant lookout for evidence of macrovascular complications of diabetes"

"Symptoms and signs of peripheral vascular disease should be sought to enable early detection and treatment"

glycaemic control and management of dyslipidaemia all reduce, postpone and possibly prevent renal and cardiovascular complications in patients with diabetes mellitus. Management of patients with diabetes in clinical practice therefore requires careful attention to multiple risk factor modification through a combination of lifestyle and pharmacological strategies.

> 66 *Management of patients with diabetes in clinical practice requires careful attention to multiple risk factor modification* 99

Dyslipidaemia

In general high concentrations of serum total cholesterol, LDL and triglycerides, and low concentrations of serum HDL confer an increased risk of CAD. The first demonstration of a link between blood cholesterol concentrations and CAD was established long ago in the Framingham Study, which demonstrated that individuals with high serum cholesterol concentrations had a several-fold increased risk of developing CAD compared with those with average concentrations.[21] Accumulated clinical trial evidence unequivocally shows that reduction of plasma cholesterol concentrations confers a significant improvement in clinical outcomes in individuals who are at high risk of cardiovascular disease.

> 66 *Reduction of plasma cholesterol concentrations confers a significant improvement in clinical outcomes in individuals who are at high risk of cardiovascular disease* 99

1994 was the beginning of a new era in lipid management as the acceptance of benefits from cholesterol lowering became more widespread. Before 1994, the first generation of lipid-lowering trials used drugs such as gemfibrozil, clofibrate and cholestyramine, which were only capable of lowering total cholesterol by as little as ~10%, and were frequently associated with adverse effects and poor compliance.[234–236] Furthermore these early studies were inadequately powered to provide a reliable estimate of the effects of lipid lowering on cardiovascular mortality. An overview of these early trials indicated that the gains in coronary heart disease reduction were related to the degree of lipid lowering and to the duration of treatment.[237] Nonetheless, the medical community was slow to adopt lipid-lowering treatment as a means of cardiovascular disease prevention, which was unlike the more general willingness to use pharmacological treatment for hypertension at the time.

> 66 *The medical community was slow to adopt lipid-lowering treatment as a means of cardiovascular disease prevention* 99

The situation changed dramatically in 1994 following publication of the 4S study, which was the first clear demonstration that choles-terol lowering as a pharmacological strategy conferred a substantially improved cardiovascular outcome in high-risk patients.[50] Since then a large number of randomized clinical trials have amassed an impressive portfolio of clinical endpoint data, now involving tens of thousands of patients. These have firmly established the benefit of pharmacological inhibition of 3-hydroxy-3-methylglutaryl coenzyme A (HMG-CoA) reductase with statin drugs for preventing fatal and non-fatal cardiovascular events.[50–54,85,86,238,239] Results of other studies have shown improved cardiovascular outcomes with non-pharmacological lipid lowering and with fibrate derivatives.[240,241] Thus there can no longer be any doubt that dyslipidaemia is a major independent risk factor for coronary heart disease and that lipid-lowering treatment saves lives and money when administered to appropriate patients. Furthermore evidence is emerging for a causal association between dyslipidaemia and increased rates of cerebrovascular disease, with clinical trial evidence suggesting reductions in stroke rates associated with statin use.[242–244] Importantly, large statin trials have shown no evidence of increased non-cardiovascular mortality.[245] Thus the benefit of treating dyslipidaemia as a means of cardiovascular risk reduction has gradually become established into clinical practice.

> *"Lipid-lowering treatment saves lives and money when administered to appropriate patients"*

Dyslipidaemia and cardiovascular risk

The MRFIT study found a strong positive association between total cholesterol concentrations and CAD risk in unselected men.[246] Moreover high cholesterol concentrations conferred a substantial increase in risk in those men who possessed additional major risk factors. Similar findings were reported in the men and women who participated in the SHEP study, which showed that lipoprotein concentrations greater than 40 mg/dL were associated with a fourfold increased CAD risk in this high-risk population.[247]

> *"Alteration of blood lipid profile, by diet or drug intervention, can successfully decrease the progression of atherosclerosis"*

Data indicate that alteration of blood lipid profile, by diet or drug intervention, can successfully decrease the progression of atherosclerosis. The degree of benefit is greatest in those with other major CAD risk factors such as hypertension, diabetes and smoking.[248] However, many patients at high risk for CAD are not achieving or maintaining recommended target lipid concentrations.[28]

Prevalence of dyslipidaemia

In 1998 the Health Survey for England and the Scottish Health Survey included representative cholesterol results for 9631 (England) and 6065 (Scotland) adults aged 16–74.[249] Mean blood levels of total cholesterol in men and women were 5.43 and 5.48 mmol/L, respectively, and HDL-cholesterol concentrations were 1.29 and 1.56 mmol/L, respectively. Overall 64.6% of adults had total cholesterol ≥5 mmol/L, 24.6% had a total:HDL ratio ≥5, and only 2.3% of the study population reported taking lipid-lowering drugs. Treatment rates among those with a total cholesterol >5 mmol/L and a clinical history of coronary heart disease or stroke, hypertension, or diabetes were 27.3%, 15.4% and 17.8%, respectively, and target total cholesterol <5 mmol/L was achieved in 45.3%, 38.5% and 32.7% of those treated, respectively.[249]

> *"Many patients at high risk for CAD are not achieving or maintaining recommended target lipid concentrations"*

Fig. 39 Prevalence of dyslipidaemia in adult men and women. TC = total cholesterol. Data from Department of Health. Health Survey for England 2003. London: The Stationery Office, 2004.

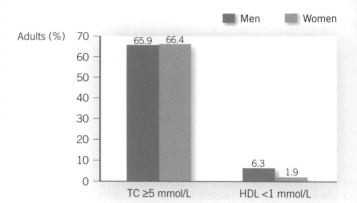

Similarly high prevalence rates of dyslipidaemia have been reported elsewhere:[250]

- moderate dyslipidaemia (total cholesterol 5.2–6.1 mmol/L) affects 30% of men and 27% of women
- severe dyslipidaemia (total cholesterol >6.2 mmol/L) affects 18% of men and 17% of women.

The prevalence of dyslipidaemia increases with advancing age, with a higher proportion of older people having raised cholesterol concentrations.

Definition and diagnosis of dyslipidaemia

As with many other CAD risk factors there appears to be a continuous relationship between cholesterol concentrations and overall risk. Therefore the cut-off points used to define the need for treatment are based on those individuals in whom their lipid profile confers a significantly high CAD risk. Meta-analysis of cohort studies shows that a 10% increase in plasma cholesterol concentration is accompanied by a 27% increase in CAD risk. Moreover a 10% reduction in cholesterol lowering by diet, drugs or surgery, conferred a 25% reduction in subsequent CAD risk after 5 years.[237]

Routine screening for dyslipidaemia should be considered for the categories of subjects summarized in Figure 40. For patients with 10-year cardiovascular disease risk less than 5% in whom total cholesterol is ≥5 mmol/L lifestyle advice is appropriate with follow-up at least every 5 years. Patients who have a 10-year cardiovascular disease risk of 5% or more, and who have total cholesterol ≥5 mmol/L, should be encouraged to follow lifestyle advice for at least 3 months. If lifestyle advice alone is insufficient then drug therapy should be contemplated to achieve target total cholesterol <5 mmol/L and LDL-cholesterol <3 mmol/L. In certain patients who have a persisting 10-year cardiovascular risk of more than

❝ There appears to be a continuous relationship between cholesterol concentrations and overall risk ❞

- men over age 40 years
- women over age 50 years
- adults with 2 risk factors for coronary heart disease (CHD)
- patients with clinical evidence of CHD, peripheral vascular disease (PVD), or carotid atherosclerosis
- patients with diabetes mellitus
- patients with xanthomata or other stigmata of dyslipidaemia
- patients with a family history of dyslipidaemia or CAD

5%, even lower target values of total cholesterol <4.5 mmol/L and LDL-cholesterol <2.5 mmol/L should be considered. Therefore using the JBS-2 risk-scoring system, a male patient aged more than 40 years with hypertension is likely to be a candidate for statin therapy based on having multiple risk factors and 10-year cardiovascular risk >5%.

Fig. 40 Assessment of lipid profile should be considered in patients in any of these categories.

Overall lifestyle measures are appropriate initial management for patients at moderate risk, in whom drug therapy should be contemplated after 3 months or more. However in patients who are at high or very high risk, drug therapy should be considered for immediate initiation. For example people with clinically evident cardiovascular disease or diabetes require aggressive LDL-cholesterol lowering to achieve total:HDL cholesterol ratio targets and reduced overall cardiovascular risk.

Reducing the risk

The cardiovascular benefits of statins were observed in studies of primary prevention of cardiovascular events in subjects with multiple risk factors and elevated plasma concentrations of LDL-cholesterol.[85] Highly positive results were also seen in studies of secondary prevention of cardiovascular events in subjects with markedly elevated LDL-cholesterol, moderately elevated LDL-cholesterol, and relatively "normal" LDL-cholesterol.[52,53,238] The landmark Heart Protection Study (HPS) enrolled subjects across a wide range of demographic and clinical characteristics and showed that lipid lowering consistently reduced cardiovascular endpoints in all subgroups irrespective of age, sex, baseline lipid profile, or presence of co-morbid conditions such as diabetes or hypertension. The HPS showed that a 1 mmol/L reduction in LDL-cholesterol with statin therapy conferred a similar benefit whether baseline concentrations were 3, 4 or 5 mmol/L.[54] The benefits extended to high-risk subjects whose pre-treatment LDL-cholesterol concentrations were already at defined "target levels", suggesting that earlier targets may not be appropriate for individuals at risk of CAD.

66In patients who are at high or very high risk, drug therapy should be considered for immediate initiation 99

The recent PROSPER study has confirmed the benefits of lipid lowering in the elderly.[86] Also, initiation of aggressive lipid-lowering early in the course of acute coronary syndromes substantially improved clinical cardiovascular outcomes and reduced the risk of stroke.[251] In addition to the impressive and consistent associations with improved clinical outcomes, these studies also confirm that statins, as a class, are safe if used properly and, in appropriately selected patients, have a potentially large benefit-to-risk ratio. A summary of factors that might influence the choice of lipid-lowering therapy is shown in Figure 41.

> *Statins, as a class, are safe if used properly and, in appropriately selected patients, have a potentially large benefit-to-risk ratio*

Relationship between lipid lowering and CAD risk reduction

In observational studies, plotting of CAD risk on a doubling scale against serum cholesterol was roughly linear, meaning that a long-term reduction in total or LDL-cholesterol concentration by ~1.0 mmol/L corresponded to ~50% less CAD, irrespective of baseline lipoproteins.[23,252] However the data are somewhat different when extrapolated from clinical trials, where reduction in risk between secondary and primary prevention appears to be different (Figure 42).[253] Generally the evidence from clinical trials has indicated that total or LDL-cholesterol lowering by 1.0 mmol/L maintained over a period of 5 years corresponds to ~35% fewer CAD events.[254]

Target lipid concentrations

Fig. 41 Selection strategy for pharmacological agents used to treat dyslipidaemia.

Target lipid concentrations are determined according to the individual's level of risk. In general targets are for total cholesterol <5 mmol/L and LDL-cholesterol <3 mmol/L as a result of lifestyle

Lipid profile	Drug of choice
Elevated LDL-cholesterol level - alone	Statin, with or without a resin or cholesterol absorption inhibitor
- with moderately elevated triglyceride	Statin, with or without a cholesterol absorption inhibitor
- with a low HDL-cholesterol	Statin, with or without a fibrate, resin, or cholesterol absorption inhibitor
	Consider niacin also
Normal LDL-cholesterol level - with an elevated triglyceride level	Niacin or fibrate or combination therapy Consider statin monotherapy if triglycerides <4 mmol/L
- with a low HDL-cholesterol level	Niacin or fibrate or combination therapy Consider statin monotherapy if triglycerides <4 mmol/L

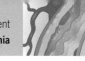

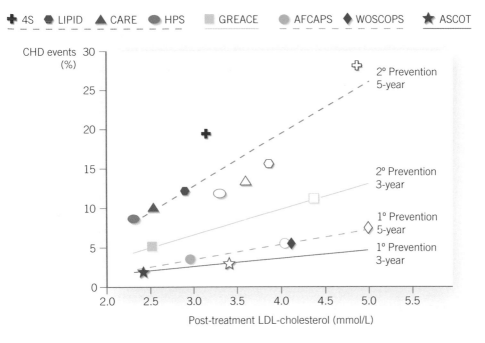

Fig. 42 Relationship between CAD events and LDL-cholesterol in recent statin trials. The filled marker is the drug treatment group, and the open marker of matching symbol is placebo or usual care group from the same study. Adapted with permission from Yusuf S, Anand S. Cost of prevention. The case of lipid lowering. Circulation 1996;93:1774–1776.

intervention with or without pharmacological intervention. In patients with established cardiovascular disease or diabetes, targets are lower for total cholesterol (<4.5 mmol/L) and LDL-cholesterol (<2.5 mmol/L) in view of their substantially increased risk.

Furthermore patients with baseline total cholesterol and LDL-cholesterol concentrations around 5 and 3 mmol/L, respectively, appear to benefit from cholesterol reduction, and treatment to lower target values of 4.5 and 2.5 mmol/L, respectively, should be considered in this group.

General principles of treatment

The management of dyslipidaemia comprises both lifestyle modification and pharmacotherapy. In contrast to the modest effects of lifestyle interventions alone, drug treatment is highly effective in favourably altering lipid profile. In high-risk patients, for example those with diabetes, it might be appropriate to initiate both lifestyle measures and pharmacotherapy simultaneously. Whereas, in individuals at lower risk, it may be appropriate to assess the effects of lifestyle modification before contemplating pharmacotherapy.

Some authorities had previously advocated improving glycaemic control in patients with diabetes, as a means of favourably modifying lipid profile, before consideration of lipid-lowering drugs. More recent

66Drug treatment is highly effective in favourably altering lipid profile 99

71

evidence suggests that, even in the presence of very poorly controlled blood glucose concentrations, improved glycaemic control might have only a modest effect on triglyceride concentrations. It is important that initiation of appropriate lipid-modifying drugs should not be withheld, especially in patients with diabetes, who are at high risk.

Pharmacological therapies

There is an increasing body of evidence in both primary and secondary prevention studies that lowering LDL concentrations with statins can reduce both cardiovascular morbidity and mortality rates in the general population.[85,255,256] The Helsinki Heart Study showed decreased cardiovascular morbidity in a primary prevention mixed dyslipidaemic population.[257] The VA-HIT trial showed decreased cardiovascular morbidity and mortality rates in a secondary prevention population characterized primarily by a low HDL treated with a fibrate.[258]

Major clinical trials carried out in the 1990s have revealed that the reduction of LDL-cholesterol concentrations with statins lowers CAD events and total mortality.[50,85,86,239] One of the more effective statins, such as simvastatin, atorvastatin or rosuvastatin, is usually required to achieve the LDL target of <2.5 mmol/L. A newer agent, ezetimibe, inhibits absorption of cholesterol in the small intestine providing a complementary action to statins. As such it can provide additional LDL-lowering when used in combination with statins and assist in reaching LDL targets. Alternatively it can provide an LDL-lowering option in patients who cannot take statins.

Fibrates are a more appropriate choice of therapy when treating high triglyceride and/or low HDL concentrations. Statins are the primary therapy for elevated LDL-cholesterol levels, while niacin or fibrates are primarily indicated for elevated triglyceride levels or low HDL-cholesterol levels. Often a single drug will be insufficient to optimize lipid concentrations in the diabetic individual. For example, a statin, even at a high dose, may lower LDL concentrations to target, but triglyceride and HDL concentrations may remain suboptimal. Similarly the use of a fibrate may be associated with improved triglyceride and HDL concentrations but suboptimal LDL concentrations. If neither class of drug alone has been demonstrated to bring all lipid concentrations to target, the combination of a statin and a fibrate can be considered, especially in patients with known vascular disease. Caution and close monitoring are required if statins are co-prescribed with fibrates due to the increased risk of myopathy and other potentially serious adverse effects. For patients receiving combined therapy, creatinine kinase concentrations should be monitored regularly and patients should be advised to stop the

❝ In individuals at lower risk, it may be appropriate to assess the effects of lifestyle modification before contemplating pharmacotherapy ❞

❝ One of the more effective statins, such as simvastatin, atorvastatin or rosuvastatin, is usually required to achieve the LDL target of <2.5 mmol/L ❞

❝ Niacin or fibrates are primarily indicated for elevated triglyceride levels or low HDL-cholesterol levels ❞

medications and inform their physician if they develop diffuse muscle aches or weakness.

Dyslipidaemia in diabetes

Although the prevalence of dyslipidaemia depends upon the definition used, dyslipidaemia is present in as many as 50% of patients with diabetes. Patients with diabetes are at particularly high risk of cardiovascular disease; for example patients with diabetes have a risk of MI similar to that in patients with established coronary disease.[259] Diabetes is associated with a two- to fivefold increased risk of cardiovascular disease, a two- to threefold increased risk of cerebrovascular disease, and a 25-fold increased risk of peripheral arterial disease. Dyslipidaemia is a major contributor to increased cardiovascular risk within this patient population, and high LDL concentrations predict an increased risk of macrovascular disease, nephropathy and retinopathy. Recognized lipid abnormalities in diabetes include:

- qualitative abnormalities in LDL (favouring oxidized state)
- low HDL-cholesterol concentrations
- high triglyceride concentrations
- increased production of very low-density lipoprotein (VLDL) by the liver in response to excess free fatty acids delivered from peripheral adipocytes
- decreased VLDL catabolism due to impaired lipoprotein lipase activity.

Although LDL-cholesterol concentrations, on average, are not increased in patients with diabetes, the LDL is more likely to be oxidized and glycosylated, both of which are thought to increase its atherogenic potential. The development of proteinuria and impaired renal function associated with the onset of diabetic nephropathy can further aggravate dyslipidaemia.

Analyses of diabetic subpopulations of large clinical studies have shown at least similar relative risk reductions in the diabetic subsets treated with lipid-lowering therapy. Therefore, given the increased cardiovascular risk in this patient group, treatment achieves a greater absolute risk reduction. The DAIS study showed a 22% decrease in angiographic measurements of focal atherosclerosis in a diabetic cohort treated with fenofibrate.[260] On the basis of all of these observations, aggressive treatment of dyslipidaemia is recommended for patients with diabetes.

All patients with diabetes should have their baseline lipid profile measured at the time of diagnosis to assist with cardiovascular risk assessment and identify the need for risk factor intervention: in order to properly assess risk, total cholesterol, LDL, HDL and triglyceride

"Caution and close monitoring are required if statins are co-prescribed with fibrates"

"High LDL concentrations predict an increased risk of macrovascular disease, nephropathy and retinopathy"

"Given the increased cardiovascular risk in this patient group, treatment achieves a greater absolute risk reduction"

concentrations should be assessed. It is especially important in this high-risk patient subgroup that target lipid concentrations are achieved through aggressive treatment and monitoring.

66 *Aggressive treatment of dyslipidaemia is recommended for patients with diabetes* 99

Can statins prevent complications of insulin resistance?

Diabetes represents a late stage of the insulin resistance syndrome, a stage at which glycaemia escapes control despite elevated serum insulin in subjects with insulin resistance. There is emerging evidence that intervening upon metabolic disturbances related to diabetes, such as dyslipidaemia, may prevent the onset of diabetes. The link between diabetes and plasma lipids was highlighted by a subgroup analysis of the WOSCOPS trial.[261] Freeman and colleagues used the 1997 American Diabetes Association diagnostic criteria to monitor the development of diabetes over 4 to 6 years in 5974 middle-aged men with no previous history of diabetes or CAD. The authors found that statin therapy was associated with a significantly lower risk of developing diabetes, with a multivariate hazard ratio of 0.70 (95% CI 0.50–0.99) compared with placebo over 4.9 years of follow-up.[261] Three possible mechanisms were suggested. First, because elevated triglycerides are associated with higher risk for development of diabetes, the known triglyceride-lowering effect of statin therapy may have been an important factor contributing to the reduced risk of diabetes. Second, several members of the statin class have been shown to have anti-inflammatory properties, which might have a beneficial influence on some of the cytokines and other inflammatory factors that promote insulin resistance. Finally, a statin-mediated improvement in endothelial function might have influenced selective tissue perfusion and thereby preserved normal glucose and insulin transport. However, other large prospective clinical trials of statin therapy have been unable to reproduce the effect on new-onset diabetes seen in the WOSCOPS trial.[54]

66 *There is emerging evidence that intervening upon metabolic disturbances related to diabetes, such as dyslipidaemia, may prevent the onset of diabetes* 99

66 *Several members of the statin class have been shown to have anti-inflammatory properties* 99

How do blood pressure measurements affect lipid targets?

Even before the availability of specific clinical trials to address the issue of intensity of lipid management in hypertensive subjects, there had been broad agreement that statin treatment should be targeted at absolute CAD risk. However there was no clear consensus on the level of risk to target. To address this issue the implications of various treatment policies to manage hypertensive patients have been examined.[262] From National Health Survey data, the proportion of hypertensive patients requiring statin treatment was at least 27%.

A sense of the benefit of combining antihypertensive and lipid-lowering treatment in hypertensive subjects was obtained from a retrospective cross-sectional study of 146 men and 150 women surveyed from general practices in Manchester, England.[263] The mean age of study subjects was 60 years, mean blood pressure was 176/102 and 176/98 mmHg in men and women, respectively, and mean serum cholesterol was 5.7 and 6.3 mmol/L in men and women, respectively. The effect of these risk factors gave the combined group a median CAD risk of 19.7% and stroke risk of 8.8% over the next 10 years. All patients received antihypertensive medication and 15% subsequently received statin treatment. On antihypertensive treatment alone, the 10-year CAD risk decreased to 16.5%. Had statin treatment been given instead, risk would have been reduced to 13.2%, based on the data from large trials. For stroke, the calculated 10-year risk on antihypertensive therapy was 5.5%, and on statin alone it was 6.2%. The study concluded that overall cardiovascular risk would be reduced from 29.4% to 22.4% by antihypertensive therapy alone and to 20.1% on a statin alone, and the effects of both treatments were statistically different (p<0.0001).[264] The authors concluded that because drug treatment in moderate hypertension is meant to reduce cardiovascular risk (and not simply to decrease blood pressure), current recommendations and practice should favour a more holistic approach, including cholesterol-lowering therapy in patients with hypertension. Meta-analyses of large clinical trials suggest that statin therapy alone might be more effective than antihypertensive therapy for reducing CAD risk, whereas antihypertensive therapy appears more effective in reducing stroke risk.[264,265] In clinical practice, using both treatments together in patients with hypertension would be expected to have even greater benefits for cardiovascular disease prevention. The benefits of statin therapy on stroke risk are shown in Figure 43.[266] It has long been recognized that in order to significantly lower cardiovascular risk, both antihypertensive and lipid-lowering therapy are needed in patients with hypertension.[267]

"Because drug treatment in moderate hypertension is meant to reduce cardiovascular risk (and not simply to decrease blood pressure), current recommendations and practice should favour a more holistic approach"

Clinical trials of lipid-lowering in hypertension

Most cardiovascular events and deaths attributable to raised blood pressure and dyslipidaemia occur among patients with blood pressure and lipid concentrations that have been traditionally considered to be "normal."[252,253] Therefore lipid-lowering therapy is important even in patients who have adequately controlled blood pressure and normal or only mildly raised plasma cholesterol. The clinical effectiveness of treating lipids among patients with elevated blood pressure has been recently evaluated in two clinical trials, namely ALLHAT and ASCOT-LLA.[268-271]

"Meta-analyses of large clinical trials suggest that statin therapy alone might be more effective than antihypertensive therapy for reducing CAD risk"

Trial, Drug	No. patients, Age range (years)	Baseline TC (mmol/L), Other	Primary endpoint, Follow-up (years)	Stroke rate (%)			Risk reduction (%)	
				Control	Statin	P value	Absolute	Relative
4S, Simvastatin	4444, 35–70	5.5–8.0	Total mortality, 5.4	4.3	2.7	0.024	1.6	30 [4–48]
CARE, Pravastatin	4159, 31–75	<6.2	CAD events, 5.0	3.8	2.6	0.03	1.2	31 [3–52]
LIPID, Pravastatin	9014, 31–75	4.0–7.0	CAD mortality, 6.0	4.5	3.7	0.048	0.8	19 [0–34]
HPS, Simvastatin	20,536, 40–80	<3.5, High-risk hyper-tensive	Total mortality, 5.3	5.7	4.3	<0.0001	1.4	25 [15–34]
PROSPER, Pravastatin	5804, 70–82	4.0–9.0, High-risk elderly	CAD death, non-fatal MI, stroke, 3.2	4.5	4.7	0.81	(0.2)	3 [-19–+31]
ALLHAT-LLT, Pravastatin	10,355, >55	3.1–4.9 or 2.6–3.3 if CAD, Hyper-tension	All-cause mortality, 4.8	4.5	4.1	0.31	0.4	9 [-25–+9]
ASCOT-LLA, Atorvastatin	10,305, 40–79	<6.5, High-risk hyper-tensive	CAD death, non-fatal MI, 3.3	2.4	1.7	0.024	0.7	27 [4–44]
GREACE, Atorvastatin	1600, <75	>2.6, Prior CAD	Total & coronary mortality, CAD events, stroke, 3.0	2.1	1.1	0.034	1.0	47
KLIS, Pravastatin	3853, 45–74	>5.6	CAD events, 5.0	2.5	2.1	0.13 (one-sided)	0.4	22 [-46–+13]
Combined data	70,070			4.32	3.44		0.9	21

Fig. 43 The effect of statin therapy on stroke risk in selected long-term statin trials and combined data.
Reproduced with permission from Amarenco P, Tonkin AM. Statins for stroke prevention: disappointment and hope. Circulation 2004;109(Suppl 1):44–49. ©American Heart Association

ALLHAT

ALLHAT was the first study with a lipid-lowering component that was performed specifically in hypertensive patients. Cardiovascular outcomes were studied in 33,357 patients aged 55 and older with hypertension and at least one additional cardiovascular risk factor. A subgroup of 10,355 patients was randomly assigned to receive either pravastatin 40 mg or usual care with respect to plasma lipoproteins. The sample was ~50% women and the mean duration of treatment was 4.8 years. Despite a 17% reduction in total serum cholesterol from baseline to year 4 in the pravastatin group, ALLHAT-LLT showed no reduction in either the primary outcome of all-cause mortality or of the secondary outcomes of non-fatal MI, stroke events, or fatal CAD compared with the placebo arm. The apparently disappointing results in ALLHAT-LLT could simply be interpreted as being consistent with the dose-response effect on cardiovascular events associated with the very modest LDL-cholesterol reduction achieved.[268,269] The apparent benefits of pravastatin might have been minimized by the prevalent use of statins in the "usual-care" group, which produced between-group differences in total and LDL cholesterol of only 9% and 17%, respectively. As few as 70% of patients in the pravastatin arm were still receiving active treatment at the end of the trial, and almost 30% in the usual-care group were given active lipid-lowering therapy. The mean difference in serum cholesterol concentration between both groups during the trial was only ~0.5 mmol/L. See Figure 44 for further details.

Nonetheless, the results of ALLHAT-LLT appeared to contradict the expectations from subgroups of patients with hypertension included in earlier statin trials. Furthermore, the findings were at odds with the PROSPER trial, which examined the benefits of pravastatin therapy in an elderly cohort of 5800 men and women with, or at a high-risk of developing, CAD and stroke.[86] In this study, pravastatin had lowered LDL-cholesterol by a more impressive 34%, which was associated with a significant reduction in the study endpoint (death from CAD, non-fatal MI, and fatal/non-fatal stroke) versus placebo.

❝The apparent benefits of pravastatin might have been minimized by the prevalent use of statins in the 'usual-care' group❞

❝The results of ALLHAT-LLT appeared to contradict the expectations from subgroups of patients with hypertension included in earlier statin trials❞

Outcome	Treatment arm	
	Pravastatin	Usual care
Reduction in total cholesterol	17.2%	7.6%
Reduction in LDL-cholesterol	27.7%	11.0%
Mortality (all causes)[1]	14.9%	15.3%
Coronary heart disease events[2]	9.3%	10.4%

Fig. 44 Results from ALLHAT lipid-lowering study.[268] [1]Relative risk 0.99; 95% CI 0.89–1.11; p=0.88, [2]Relative risk 0.91; 95% CI 0.79–1.04; p=0.16.

The ALLHAT-LLT study might have failed to demonstrate a benefit from pravastatin therapy because the differences in achieved cholesterol concentrations were less impressive than in the PROSPER trial. In order to achieve target LDL-cholesterol of <2.5 mmol/L in clinical practice, pharmacological management generally requires use of a statin that is more efficacious (e.g. atorvastatin, simvastatin or rosuvastatin).

> *" In order to achieve target LDL-cholesterol of <2.5 mmol/L in clinical practice, pharmacological management generally requires use of a statin that is more efficacious "*

ASCOT-LLA

ASCOT was an investigator-initiated and led, multicentre, randomized trial designed to compare two antihypertensive strategies in more than 19,000 patients.[270,271] A lipid-lowering arm (ASCOT-LLA) assessed the effects of lipid lowering on cardiovascular outcomes in patients with hypertension who had total cholesterol concentrations >6.5 mmol/L. The primary objective of ASCOT-LLA was to assess long-term effects of treatment with atorvastatin (plus antihypertensive treatment) compared with placebo (plus matched antihypertensive treatment) on the combined endpoint of non-fatal MI, including silent MI, and fatal CAD. Secondary endpoints of ASCOT-LLA were the primary outcome without silent events, all-cause mortality, total cardiovascular mortality, fatal and non-fatal stroke, fatal and non-fatal heart failure, total coronary endpoints, and total cardiovascular events. Tertiary objectives included the assessment of the effects of statin on the primary endpoint among several subgroups. Of the total 19,342 patients with hypertension, 10,305 were randomized to receive atorvastatin 10 mg or placebo. The study population was mostly male, elderly and had an average of 3.7 risk factors in addition to hypertension and, therefore, was a high-risk population. Eighty-seven per cent of the patients originally assigned atorvastatin were still taking it at trial end, and only 9% of those on placebo had been prescribed open-label statin treatment.

> *" ASCOT-LLA ended prematurely at 3.3 years because an interim analysis showed a significant benefit of atorvastatin treatment "*

The planned 5-year follow-up in ASCOT-LLA ended prematurely at 3.3 years because an interim analysis showed a significant benefit of atorvastatin treatment. Specifically, by that time-point 100 primary events had occurred in the atorvastatin group (n=5168) compared with 154 in the placebo group (n=5137), representing a relative risk reduction of 36% (HR 0.64, 95% CI 0.50–0.83, p=0.0005). This benefit was clearly seen to emerge within the first year of follow-up. There were significant reductions in other pre-specified outcomes, such as fatal and non-fatal stroke (89 atorvastatin versus 121 placebo, HR 0.73, 95% CI 0.56–0.96, p=0.024) and total cardiovascular events (389 atorvastatin versus 486 placebo, HR 0.79, 95% CI 0.69–0.90, p=0.0005).

Atorvastatin lowered total serum cholesterol by a net ~1.3 mmol/L compared with placebo at 12 months, and by a net ~1.1 mmol/L after 3 years of follow-up. The ASCOT-LLA investigators estimated that event reduction would have approached 50% if the study had continued for 5 years and had not been terminated early. A mean reduction in total cholesterol of ~1.0 mmol/L is consistent with a 50% reduction in events over 5 years, based on observational studies of serum cholesterol.

ASCOT-LLA in the context of other statin trials

Before the widespread use of statins, epidemiological studies suggested only a weak relationship between serum total cholesterol concentrations and stroke risk.[243] However early large trials of statin therapy consistently showed reductions in stroke events in both primary and secondary prevention ranging from 15% to 30%.[244] The findings from ASCOT-LLA replicated and extended the findings of earlier clinical trials of statins. After 1 year of follow-up in ASCOT-LLA, total and LDL-cholesterol among patients taking atorvastatin were 24% and 35% lower, respectively, than in patients receiving placebo. By comparison, in the WOSCOPS study, 40 mg pravastatin reduced total and LDL-cholesterol by only 20% and 26%, respectively, which was associated with a reduction in non-fatal MI and fatal CAD of 31% after 4.9 years of follow-up.[239] In AFCAPS/TexCAPS statin treatment reduced total and LDL-cholesterol by 18% and 25%, respectively, which was associated with a reduction in non-fatal MI and fatal CAD of 40% after 4.2 years of follow-up.[85] These degrees of event reduction seen in the various trials, including ASCOT-LLA, are thus very comparable given the magnitude of LDL lowering afforded by specific treatments and trial duration.

Surprisingly, and in contrast with other statin trials involving high-risk patient subgroups, the ASCOT-LLA did not find any significant treatment effect in the subgroup of 2532 patients with diabetes. However the absolute number of events among patients with diabetes was only 84 and the apparent absence of event reduction probably reflected inadequate statistical power, especially given the shortened follow-up period. This could also have been related to higher open-label use of statins in the placebo arm among patients with diabetes versus those without diabetes (14% versus 8%, respectively). In ASCOT-LLA the 27% reduction in stroke incidence was similar in magnitude to the effect of statin therapy observed in other large lipid-lowering trials. One notable exception was the PROSPER trial[86] of pravastatin administered to patients aged 70 years and older, which reported no reduction in strokes. Interestingly, a post hoc analysis of 2416 patients older than 70 years in ASCOT-LLA showed similar

"The ASCOT-LLA investigators estimated that event reduction would have approached 50% if the study had continued for 5 years"

"Early large trials of statin therapy consistently showed reductions in stroke events"

atorvastatin-related stroke reduction compared with subjects aged 70 years or younger (31% versus 24% reduction, respectively).

While the results of ASCOT-LLA were exciting, consideration needs to be given to the resource implications of widespread statin use among all hypertensive patients with absolute levels of cardiovascular risk similar to those included in ASCOT. There were large relative reductions in cardiovascular events associated with statin use in hypertensive patients who were at only moderate cardiovascular risk and did not have dyslipidaemia according to conventional criteria. The wider benefits of statin therapy in hypertensive patients remain to be seen, and the 36% relative reduction in the primary endpoint observed in ASCOT needs to be weighed against the fact that the absolute risk reduction of a coronary event was 3.4 per 1000 patient-years.

Do the ASCOT-LLA results change the threshold for statin treatment?

The placebo group in ASCOT-LLA had a 9.4% 10-year coronary event rate (non-fatal MI and fatal CAD) and a 7.4% 10-year fatal and non-fatal stroke event rate.[271] Thus, the combined first stroke or CAD event rate in the ASCOT-LLA sample was ~16.5%. Risk estimation that is used to decide whether to treat such patients includes measurement of blood pressure before treatment.[270] After 3 years of follow-up, mean blood pressure in the ASCOT volunteers had fallen by ~25/14 mmHg.[270] Had these subjects not received aggressive blood pressure-lowering treatment, the cardiovascular risk in the placebo group would have exceeded 20% over 10 years, which is close to the level of global cardiovascular and CAD risk that is increasingly accepted as a reasonable treatment threshold for lipid-lowering. Thus, the ASCOT-LLA results reinforce the emerging trend to adopt lower lipid-lowering treatment thresholds, at least among patients with moderate hypertension.

ALLHAT-LLT versus ASCOT-LLA

In ALLHAT-LLT the use of pravastatin versus usual care in patients with mild-to-moderate hypertension produced non-significant reductions in cardiovascular events compared with the very significant results seen in hypertensive subjects treated with atorvastatin in ASCOT-LLA. The less impressive outcomes in ALLHAT-LLT compared with ASCOT-LLA could have many possible explanations. The key difference was in the efficacy of the two statin treatments. Atorvastatin caused ~1.0 mmol/L cholesterol reduction in ASCOT-LLA, whereas pravastatin caused only a ~0.5 mmol/L reduction in ALLHAT-LLT. Also, the baseline demographics of patients included in ALLHAT-LLT were substantially different from those of patients

> *Consideration needs to be given to the resource implications of widespread statin use among all hypertensive patients with absolute levels of cardiovascular risk similar to those included in ASCOT*

> *The ASCOT-LLA results reinforce the emerging trend to adopt lower lipid-lowering treatment thresholds*

in ASCOT-LLA: ALLHAT included an older cohort, of whom about 14% had established CAD, and a notably greater proportion (~50%) were women and non-Caucasian people. There was greater adherence to statin therapy in the active study arm in ASCOT-LLA versus ALLHAT-LLT, and the prevalence of statin use in the placebo arm was lower in ASCOT-LLA. All of these factors mean that the ASCOT-LLA study was more likely to demonstrate a difference between statin and placebo-treated groups.

> **❝The baseline demographics of patients included in ALLHAT-LLT were substantially different from those of patients in ASCOT-LLA❞**

Do statins lower blood pressure directly?

There is some evidence that statins can reduce blood pressure. For instance, in small clinical investigative studies, statins have been shown to decrease systolic, diastolic and pulse pressures.[272–276] In general the improvement in blood pressure in these small studies is relatively acute and related to the extent of cholesterol lowering. However large clinical trials, on the whole, have not shown any extra benefit of statin treatment on improvement of blood pressure, and have not shown any significant blood pressure-lowering effects of statins compared with placebo. However the issue remains incompletely resolved by studies such as ASCOT, since the design included an upward titration of anti-hypertensive medication based on achieved blood pressure, thereby potentially masking any impact of statin treatment on blood pressure.

> **❝In small clinical investigative studies, statins have been shown to decrease systolic, diastolic, and pulse pressures❞**

Conclusions

Studies from across many European countries indicate that there is currently suboptimal use of lipid-lowering treatment in clinical practice.[277] The findings to date, especially in ASCOT-LLA, support the concept that treatment strategies to reduce cardiovascular disease should depend on global assessment of risk, rather than on arbitrary numerical cut-off values for individual risk factors, and that benefits of lipid lowering are apparent across the whole range of serum cholesterol concentrations. The overall benefits in terms of preventing cardiovascular events attributable to one strategy or another in any given patient depends on the demography and global CAD risk for that individual patient. For example, in northern Europe and North America, where CAD events are more common than stroke, greater overall benefits might be obtained from lipid lowering than from blood pressure lowering alone. However, the overwhelming preponderance of data show the benefits of statin treatment are additive to those of good blood pressure control. Consequently, more serious consideration now needs to be given to the most resource-effective way of providing both of these risk factor intervention strategies for hypertensive patients in order to prevent fatal and non-fatal cardiovascular events.

> **❝Treatment strategies to reduce cardiovascular disease should depend on global assessment of risk, rather than on arbitrary numerical cut-off values for individual risk factors❞**

81

Hypertension

Hypertension is one of the leading mortality risk factors worldwide, and is recognized in around one third of all global mortality, and up to half of all cardiovascular disease. In the majority of Western countries the cost of arterial hypertension absorbs a large and growing share of health resources. Hypertension is strongly and causally associated with CAD, congestive heart failure, haemorrhagic stroke, stroke, cardiovascular disease and premature death. Current estimates suggest that about 30–40% of MI, 30–40% of strokes, 25–30% of renal failure, 50% of atrial fibrillation and up to 50% of heart failure are directly attributable to hypertension. Hypertension is also associated with significant morbidity from renal failure, aortic aneurysm, peripheral vascular disease, dementia, atrial fibrillation and erectile dysfunction.[84,278–281] Clinical trials have suggested that treatment of ISH can prevent development or progression of dementia, which requires confirmation in specific prospective studies.[279] Most patients with hypertension have multiple other risk factors for cardiovascular disease. However, in most situations, it is blood pressure treatment and control that will offer the greatest overall benefit. Often hypertension is not recorded on death certificates as a secondary or contributing cause, so the true impact on health outcomes is likely to be significantly underestimated.

In 1998 around 5.7 million adults in the UK (12% of the population aged >16 years) had blood pressure higher than 160/95 mmHg, and 16 million (33%) had blood pressure greater than 140/90 mmHg.[282] High blood pressure is thought to have caused 58,000 excess major cardiovascular events per year in this population over and above the expected rate associated with blood pressure treated to target values, which represents a direct healthcare cost of almost £100 million annually.[282] Therefore failure to achieve appropriate blood pressure control confers a substantial excess cardiovascular risk, and makes a significant contribution to a potentially avoidable healthcare financial burden.

Definition of hypertension

Blood pressure is a continuously variable measurement across populations. A strong positive correlation exists between blood pressure and cardiovascular risk but it is impossible to clearly delineate "normal" from "abnormal" blood pressures. The values used in clinical practice to define hypertension have been chosen so as to allow identification of patients in whom blood pressure is sufficiently high to impose a significant increase in overall cardiovascular risk. As data have steadily accrued from large clinical trials, increasing information has emerged regarding the contribution of blood pressure to cardio-

> *Data show the benefits of statin treatment are additive to those of good blood pressure control*

> *The cost of arterial hypertension absorbs a large and growing share of health resources*

> *Failure to achieve appropriate blood pressure control confers a substantial excess cardiovascular risk*

vascular risk at progressively lower values. Therefore the cut-off blood pressure values used to diagnose hypertension have progressively fallen, and larger proportions of populations are thought to be at increased CAD risk due to high blood pressure. The current guidelines from the Joint National Committee on hypertension (JNC VII guidelines) characterize optimal systolic and diastolic blood pressures of no more than 120 and 80 mmHg, respectively, whereas pressures greater than 140 or 90 mmHg, respectively, define hypertension.[283]

It is impossible to clearly delineate 'normal' from 'abnormal' blood pressures

Prevalence of hypertension

Based on the current JNC VII criteria, hypertension is prevalent in around one in four adults in Western societies, and affects 1 billion people worldwide. Given the high prevalence of the disorder, family physicians have a particularly important role in identifying individuals with hypertension and taking steps to optimize cardiovascular risk reduction in these people. Most of the risk associated with high blood pressure can be reversed by appropriate therapy. In order to optimally reduce the burden of illness associated with hypertension, physicians need to:

- accurately assess blood pressure in high-risk patients
- identify those with, and at risk of developing, hypertension
- initiate therapy based on the individual's risk of developing cardio-vascular disease and treat their risk factors to target (Figure 45).[283]

A number of tools aim to assist physicians in achieving target blood pressures in individual patients and populations:

- regularly updated evidence-based hypertension recommendations
- tools to aid the implementation of recommendations, for example electronic risk calculators

Fig. 45 Treatment goals for hypertension, based on existing guidelines.[283]

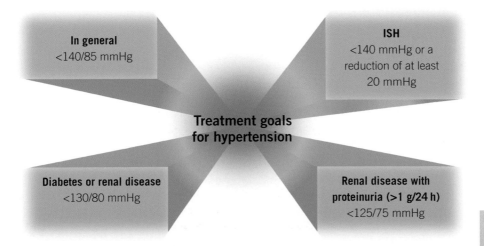

In general
<140/85 mmHg

ISH
<140 mmHg or a reduction of at least 20 mmHg

Treatment goals for hypertension

Diabetes or renal disease
<130/80 mmHg

Renal disease with proteinuria (>1 g/24 h)
<125/75 mmHg

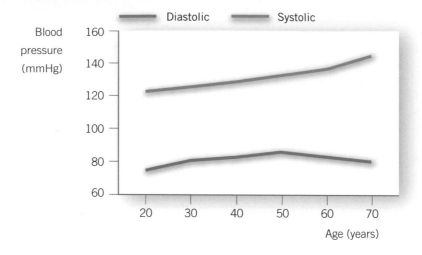

Fig. 46 Mean systolic and diastolic blood pressure values in a Western population, shown across different age groups.[286]

• increasing focus of large clinical trials on addressing clinically relevant questions related to risk reduction.

Prevalence of ISH

Elevated systolic blood pressure in the presence of normal diastolic blood pressure, so-called ISH, results in increased pulse pressure (i.e. systolic pressure minus diastolic pressure), and is an important CAD risk factor.[284–286] Historically, greater attention has focused on diastolic pressure as a risk factor and target for antihypertensive therapy. However over the past 10 years it has become known that systolic blood pressure plays a larger role than diastolic blood pressure in predicting adverse cardiovascular outcomes, particularly in elderly patients. Clinical trials demonstrating large benefits of antihypertensive drug therapy in ISH have accelerated the shift in interest away from diastolic hypertension to ISH and pulse pressure.[83,84,247] Using current definitions systolic hypertension is described by sustained clinic systolic blood pressures >140 mmHg, and diastolic hypertension defined by sustained clinic diastolic blood pressures >90 mmHg.[283] ISH is defined by average clinic systolic blood pressure >140 mmHg but where diastolic blood pressure is <90 mmHg.

Systolic blood pressure increases progressively throughout adulthood while diastolic blood pressure increases to about age 55–60 years and then decreases with age (Figure 46). The prevalence of ISH and isolated diastolic hypertension are, therefore, largely related to age. With progressively increasing age, an increasing proportion of patients will have ISH whereas a declining proportion of patients will have high diastolic blood pressure (Figure 47).[286]

> **"** Systolic blood pressure plays a larger role than diastolic blood pressure in predicting adverse cardiovascular outcomes, particularly in elderly patients **"**

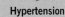

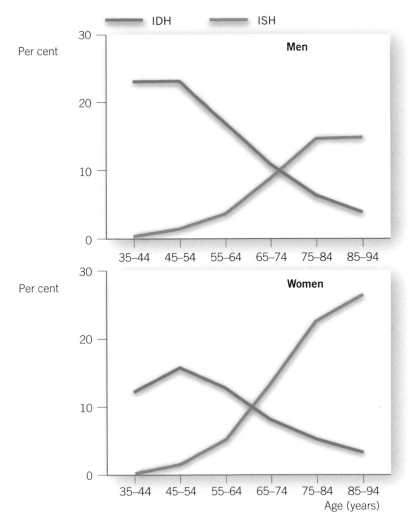

Fig. 47 Proportion of patients with hypertension that falls into the category of isolated diastolic hypertension (IDH) or isolated systolic hypertension (ISH) across different age groups.[282]

Despite widespread availability of guidelines that inform clinical practice with regard to blood pressure treatment, the prevalence of hypertension is increasing rapidly. Data from the USA, Egypt and China show that more than 25% of adults with hypertension were unaware of their diagnosis. Furthermore, only 55% of patients in the USA were receiving antihypertensive treatment, and only 29% of patients receiving antihypertensive medication had achieved target systolic and diastolic blood pressure targets of 140 and 90 mmHg or lower, respectively. In Egypt and China the proportions of adults with hypertension who were treated to systolic <140 mmHg and diastolic <90 mmHg were only 8% and <5%, respectively.[287] These data underpin

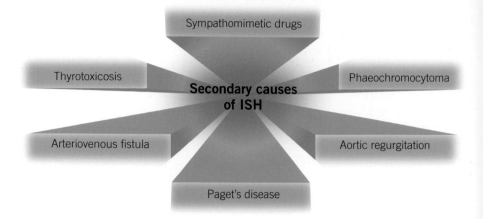

Sympathomimetic drugs

Thyrotoxicosis

Phaeochromocytoma

Secondary causes of ISH

Arteriovenous fistula

Aortic regurgitation

Paget's disease

Fig. 48 Secondary causes of ISH.

Fig. 49 Changes in cardiovascular risk associated with systolic blood pressure (SBP), in the presence of high or low diastolic blood pressure (DBP).[290]

the fact that hypertension is highly prevalent but is under-recognized and inadequately treated, particularly in developing countries.

In Western populations, ISH is prevalent in fewer than one in 20 adults aged less than 45 years, and dramatically increases to over one in three of those aged over 65 years.[288] The increase in ISH with age is even more marked in women than men. Up to half of all adults over the age of 65 years have systolic hypertension and more than one-third have ISH.[288] Risk factors for ISH are shown in Figure 48. The relationship between cardiovascular risk, and systolic and diastolic blood pressures is shown in Figure 49.[289] The relationship between diastolic pressure and risk is complex. If systolic pressure is normal, then a

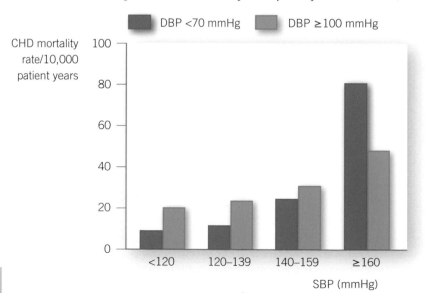

CHD mortality rate/10,000 patient years

DBP <70 mmHg   DBP ≥100 mmHg

SBP (mmHg)

positive association between diastolic pressure and cardiovascular risk emerges, especially in younger patients (Figure 50). However, if the systolic pressure is high, then a stronger inverse relationship is observed between diastolic pressure and risk, so those at highest risk are patients with ISH.[289,290] Increases in systolic and decreases in diastolic blood pressures are associated with increased risk, as indicated by increased pulse pressure (pulse pressure is the difference between systolic and diastolic blood pressure values). Consistent with the above, many studies have reported that increased pulse pressure provides additional risk prediction over and above that of systolic pressure alone.[265,266] With the current trend towards a progressively ageing population, and changes in lifestyles that increase the risk of developing systolic hypertension, it is likely that there will be substantial increases in the already staggering number of patients with ISH.

66Many studies have reported that increased pulse pressure provides additional risk prediction over and above that of systolic pressure alone 99

Measurement of blood pressure
The diagnosis of hypertension may seem straightforward, but in reality represents several challenges.[291,292] The first issue is the accurate measurement of blood pressure. If done properly measurement takes approximately 8 minutes and requires attention to patient preparation (Figure 51), measurement technique (Figure 52) and appropriate equipment. Unfortunately in clinical practice measurement of blood pressure and diagnosis are frequently done without attention to detail. One study found that the diagnosis changed for more than one in every two patients when blood pressure was measured with greater attention to detail rather than by the usual technique.[293]

Fig. 50 **Changes in cardiovascular risk associated with diastolic blood pressure (DBP), in the presence of high or low systolic blood pressure (SBP).**[290]

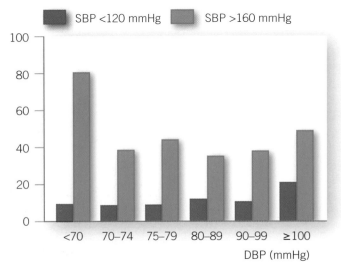

> ❝ *In clinical practice measurement of blood pressure and diagnosis are frequently done without attention to detail* ❞

Ideally blood pressure should be checked in the seated position, using the right or left arm, after the patient has rested for at least 5 minutes. Both arms should be used to assess initial blood pressure. If there is a significant difference between left and right arms, for example due to advanced atherosclerosis, then the arm that gives the highest readings should be used because this is more reflective of true blood pressure. Blood pressure should be checked after standing for 2 minutes in patients with diabetes and elderly patients in order to detect significant orthostatic hypotension. An appropriate cuff size should be used, for example a larger-sized blood pressure cuff will be required for obese patients.

Variability of blood pressure increases with age, likely related to reduced baroceptor function and reduced arterial compliance. The increased variability of blood pressure makes the diagnosis of hypertension more challenging and this can in part be addressed by more frequent measurements. This has raised important questions regarding the potential roles of patient self-measurement of blood pressure and 24-hour ambulatory blood pressure measurement (ABPM). In

Fig. 51 Factors to take into consideration when preparing to undertake blood pressure measurement.

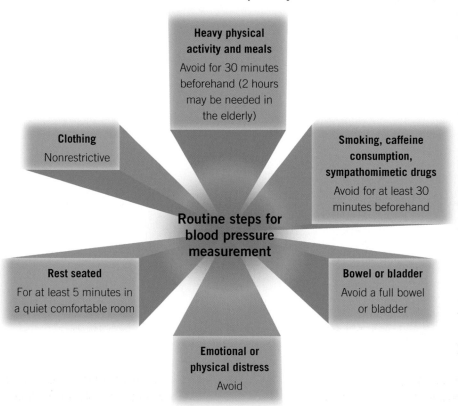

Heavy physical activity and meals
Avoid for 30 minutes beforehand (2 hours may be needed in the elderly)

Clothing
Nonrestrictive

Smoking, caffeine consumption, sympathomimetic drugs
Avoid for at least 30 minutes beforehand

Routine steps for blood pressure measurement

Rest seated
For at least 5 minutes in a quiet comfortable room

Bowel or bladder
Avoid a full bowel or bladder

Emotional or physical distress
Avoid

1. Preferably use a mercury manometer, but a recently calibrated aneroid or a validated and recently calibrated electronic device can be used. Aneroid devices and mercury columns must be clearly visible at eye level

2. Choose a cuff with an appropriate bladder width (bladder width x 2.5) +/– 4 cm = arm circumference

3. Place the cuff so that the lower edge is 3 cm above the elbow crease and the bladder is centred over the brachial artery. The patient should be resting comfortably seated with back support for 5 minutes. The arm should be bare and supported with the antecubital fossa at heart level. There should be no talking, and the patient's legs should not be crossed. (Blood pressure should also be assessed after standing for 2 minutes and at times when the patient complains of symptoms suggestive of postural hypotension)

4. Increase the pressure rapidly to 30 mmHg above the level at which the radial pulse is extinguished (to exclude the possibility of auscultatory gap)

5. Place the head of the stethoscope gently but firmly over the brachial artery

6. Open the control valve so that the rate of drop in the vicinity of the SBP and DBP is 2 mmHg per beat

7. Read the SBP – the first appearance of a clear tapping sound (phase I Korotkoff) – and the DBP, the point at which the sounds disappear (phase V Korotkoff). If Korotkoff sounds persist as the level approaches 0 mmHg, the point of muffling of the sound (phase IV) is used to indicate the DBP

8. Record:
- blood pressure to the closest 2 mmHg on the manometer (or 1 mmHg on electronic devices)
- arm used
- position (supine, sitting or standing)
- heart rate

(Seated blood pressure is used to determine and monitor treatment. Standing blood pressure is used to examine for postural hypotension, which may modify the treatment)

9. In the case of arrhythmia, additional readings may be needed to estimate the average SBP and DBP. Isolated extra beats should be ignored. Note rhythm and pulse rate

10. Leaving the cuff partially inflated for too long, fills the venous system and makes the sounds difficult to hear. To avoid venous congestion, at least 1 minute should elapse between readings

11. Blood pressure should be taken at least once in both arms; if an arm has a consistently higher pressure, it should be used subsequently

Fig. 52 Suggested technique for single measurement of blood pressure. DBP = diastolic blood pressure, SBP = systolic blood pressure. Note: patients with diabetes should be checked for significant orthostatic hypotension.

general, serial office blood pressures taken with care are thought to be as predictive of target organ damage and future outcome as ABPM.[294]

Making a clinical diagnosis of hypertension

66 A hypertensive crisis should alert the physician to the need for prompt treatment 99

A diagnosis of hypertension relates to both the presence of target organ damage and the level of blood pressure, and should be set in the context of overall cardiovascular risk.[292] A hypertensive crisis should alert the physician to the need for prompt treatment. In such cases, where hypertension may be severe with evidence of end-organ damage, assessment, diagnosis and management are more urgent. Figure 53 shows some situations where immediate diagnosis and management may be indicated. Blood pressure often decreases over several visits and, if the initial systolic blood pressure is <180 mmHg and any target organ damage appears stable, then observation over three separate visits is recommended. Assessment of blood pressure over five or more separate visits may be helpful in establishing a more representative baseline value, and should be considered for people without any clinical evidence of cardiovascular complications or target organ damage (Figure 54) and if initial systolic blood pressure is <180 mmHg. If the blood pressure is not falling, or is increasing over serial visits, then a

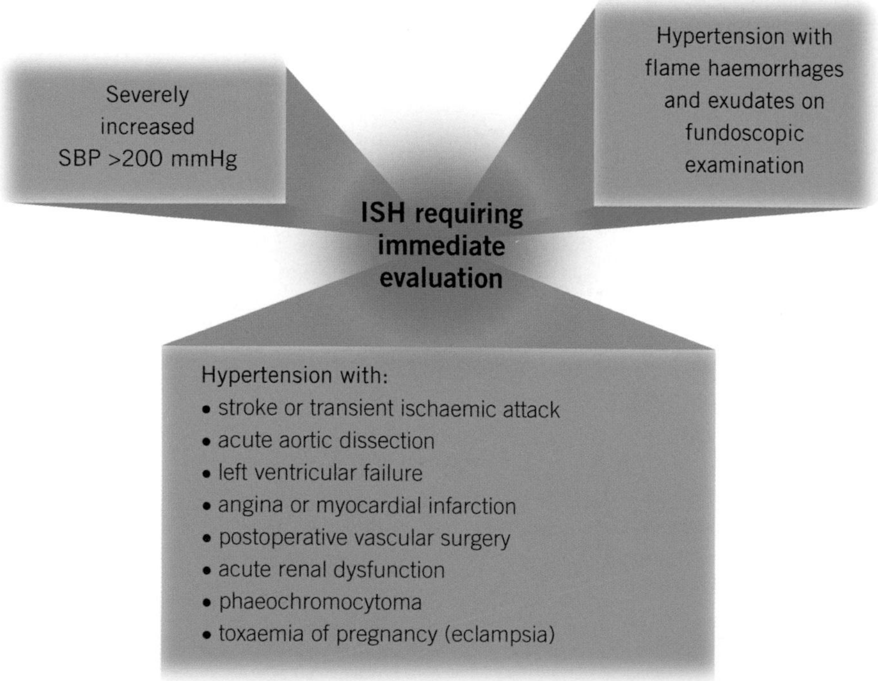

Fig. 53 Situations that should alert the physician to the need for more urgent evaluation and treatment. SBP = systolic blood pressure.

Severely increased SBP >200 mmHg

Hypertension with flame haemorrhages and exudates on fundoscopic examination

ISH requiring immediate evaluation

Hypertension with:
- stroke or transient ischaemic attack
- acute aortic dissection
- left ventricular failure
- angina or myocardial infarction
- postoperative vascular surgery
- acute renal dysfunction
- phaeochromocytoma
- toxaemia of pregnancy (eclampsia)

diagnosis of hypertension is more easy to establish, and more than three assessment visits are unlikely to be helpful. The category and severity of hypertension can be described using the guidelines issued by the British Hypertension Society (BHS, Figure 55).[295]

Self- or home measurement of blood pressure

The benefits of self-measurement of blood pressure are largely unproven. One of the more established benefits is increased adherence to antihypertensive therapy in those who are initially non-adherent.[296] In this indication, high blood pressure seems to encourage pill taking and a lower blood pressure when adherent is positive reinforcement for pill taking. Although proof of effectiveness is lacking, self-measurement can be of assistance in:

* monitoring those with white-coat hypertension
* monitoring drug therapy in patients with variable blood pressure
* assessing patient symptoms that may relate to hypotension.

There are several caveats to using self-measurement. Some patients lack the ability to self-measure blood pressure, and all patients require training specific to the equipment they use. Electronic devices have

> **"Assessment of blood pressure over five or more separate visits may be helpful in establishing a more representative baseline value"**

Fig. 54 Common examples of target organ damage.

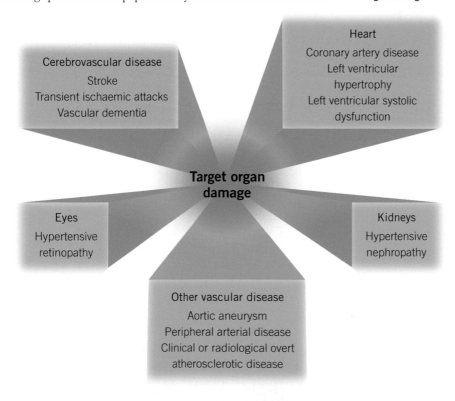

Cerebrovascular disease
Stroke
Transient ischaemic attacks
Vascular dementia

Heart
Coronary artery disease
Left ventricular hypertrophy
Left ventricular systolic dysfunction

Target organ damage

Eyes
Hypertensive retinopathy

Kidneys
Hypertensive nephropathy

Other vascular disease
Aortic aneurysm
Peripheral arterial disease
Clinical or radiological overt atherosclerotic disease

Classification of blood pressure		
Category	**Systolic blood pressure (mmHg)**	**Diastolic blood pressure (mmHg)**
Optimal blood pressure	<120	<80
Normal blood pressure	<130	<85
High-normal blood pressure	130–139	85–89
Grade 1 hypertension (mild)	140–159	90–99
Grade 2 hypertension (moderate)	160–179	100–109
Grade 3 hypertension (severe)	⩾180	⩾110
Isolated systolic hypertension (Grade 1)	140–159	<90
Isolated systolic hypertension (Grade 2)	⩾160	<90

Fig. 55 Classification of blood pressure as indicated by the most recent British Hypertension Society guidelines. Reproduced with permission from Williams B, Poulter NR, Brown MJ, et al. British Hypertension Society guidelines for hypertension management 2004 (BHS-IV): summary. BMJ 2004;328:634–640. © BMJ Publishing Group

> 66 *The interpretation of self-measured readings is difficult, but these are generally expected to be lower than office recordings* 99

some advantages in that they require less patient skill and are not dependent on patient hearing. Aneroid devices can be used by patients, but require good hearing, manual dexterity and more extensive training to establish accurate techniques. Only electronic devices meeting international standards should be recommended for use by patients. The major international standards are the BHS and the Association for the Advancement of Medical Instrumentation (AAMI).[297,298] The BHS website also lists devices that have passed standard reference criteria (http://www.bhsoc.org/blood_pressure_list.htm). Currently self-measured readings are considered a supplement to and not a replacement for office readings. The interpretation of self-measured readings is difficult, but these are generally expected to be lower than office recordings. Self-measured systolic and diastolic blood pressures of >135 mmHg and >85 mmHg, respectively, are likely to be consistent with a diagnosis of hypertension, and should be considered for therapy if the office readings are also above treatment cut-off points. If a person has hypertension in the office and normal self-measured readings, then self-measured readings may need to be confirmed using another technique such as ABPM before concluding that the person has white-coat hypertension.[299]

ABPM

ABPM is a useful technique in the diagnosis of ISH. Interpretation of readings is aided by understanding that normal mean systolic and diastolic readings are <135 mmHg and <85 mmHg during wakefulness, and <120 mmHg and <70 mmHg during sleep, respectively.[300] However it is also recognized that optimal blood pressure values are likely to be even lower, especially in high-risk patients, and optimal blood pressure values are regarded as:

- average awake ABPM systolic and diastolic blood pressure readings <130 mmHg and <88 mmHg, respectively
- average asleep systolic and diastolic blood pressures of <115 mmHg and <65 mmHg, respectively.[300]

A dip in nocturnal (asleep) blood pressure values is normal. In patients with hypertension, those who do not have a 10–20% decrease in nocturnal pressures are said to be "non-dippers", and appear to have significantly increased cardiovascular risk compared with "dippers". Nonetheless it is important to note that the results of ABPM in clinical practice are not very reproducible. In patients with white-coat hypertension or who have a non-dipping pattern, around 30–40% will have sustained hypertension with a normal nocturnal dipping pattern on retesting.[295,301] Therefore results from ABPM require confirmation by repeat testing or use of other techniques if the readings alter management decisions. The presence of white-coat hypertension indicates a risk that is intermediate between sustained hypertension and normal blood pressure. Patients require follow-up because a large proportion will develop sustained hypertension if monitored for a sufficient period of time.

> **"It is important to note that the results of ABPM in clinical practice are not very reproducible"**

Diagnostic pitfalls

There are several circumstances where the usual measurement of blood pressure can result in an erroneous diagnosis of hypertension or the false perception of normal blood pressure.

Factors that give the appearance of normal blood pressure in hypertension:

- a partially obstructed subclavian or axillary artery (e.g. due to advanced atherosclerosis) – the partial obstruction results in a blood pressure lower than systemic blood pressure in the arm with the obstruction
- measuring blood pressure in the flaccid arm after a stroke – it has been suggested that this results in a falsely low blood pressure due to reduced blood flow
- postprandial hypotension, which is more common in the elderly and is particularly common in nursing home populations – although this usually results in adverse events during therapy, measurement after meals can cause the perception that blood pressure is normal.

> **"Results from ABPM require confirmation by repeat testing or use of other techniques if the readings alter management decisions"**

Factors that cause a false perception of hypertension

One of the most common patterns in this category is "white-coat" hypertension, or "isolated clinic" hypertension. In this situation the office blood pressure readings are high, but the average blood pressure measured outside the hospital or GP clinic is normal. Confirmation and monitoring with self-measurement and ABPM are suggested for those in whom this is suspected.[300] It is important to bear in mind that the presence of white-coat hypertension on ABPM is not reproduced in up to 30–40% of patients, and that persons with white-coat hypertension appear to be at increased risk of developing sustained hypertension over time.[295] The extent to which white-coat hypertension might be associated with cardiovascular risk is uncertain. Most data would suggest that the excess risk associated with this blood pressure pattern is intermediate between sustained normal blood pressures and sustained hypertension. Therefore ongoing monitoring with self- or ambulatory monitoring is necessary in all patients with white-coat hypertension.

Factors that give the false impression of high blood pressure readings:

- pseudohypertension is thought to arise when the brachial artery is muscular and rigid and can withstand higher cuff pressures than the pressure of the blood within the vessel – the measurement of pressure using a cuff in this situation results in pressures higher than intra-arterial pressures. This is a recognized cause for falsely high blood pressure recordings particularly in healthy young males
- "in cuff" hypertension, the inflation of the blood pressure cuff transiently increases intra-arterial pressure and results in the false perception that the person has hypertension.

Both pseudohypertension and "in cuff" hypertension can be suspected if there is no target organ damage, particularly if there is a long history of hypertension. Some of those who have a false elevation of blood pressure also have symptoms of hypotension or fatigue during treatment. Measuring blood pressure in an arm with muscular spasticity (e.g. after a stroke) can also result in a falsely high estimate of systemic blood pressure because the rigid upper limb muscles prevent the brachial artery from cuff compression.

Pathogenesis of hypertension

A number of different mechanisms appear to be involved in the development and progression of hypertension, including activation of the sympathetic nervous system and renin-angiotensin-aldosterone cascade, abnormal baroreceptor function, endothelial dysfunction and high blood pressure sensitivity to salt intake. In a small proportion of cases a single pathway can be identified as a primary cause, for example renal artery stenosis or endocrine disorders including Cushing's syndrome, phaeochromocytoma or Conn's disease, and in a very small number of patients there appears to be a particularly strong genetic basis for the development of hypertension. Nonetheless in more than

> *Persons with white-coat hypertension appear to be at increased risk of developing sustained hypertension over time*

> *Ongoing monitoring with self- or ambulatory monitoring is necessary in all patients with white-coat hypertension*

> *Some of those who have a false elevation of blood pressure also have symptoms of hypotension or fatigue during treatment*

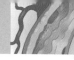

95% of patients with hypertension there is no identifiable single cause, so-called "essential" hypertension. To a greater or lesser extent, many patients with essential hypertension are found to have activation of mechanisms that contribute to sustained hypertension, including activation of the sympathetic nervous system and renin-angiotensin-aldosterone system, and impairment of endothelial function.

Regardless of the factors initiating the development of hypertension, a number of cardiac and vascular responses to high blood pressure result in functional and structural alterations that can sustain high blood pressure levels. Structural alterations to high blood pressure lead to thickening of the intima and hypertrophy of the medial layer in the vascular tree.[302,303] This eventually progresses to loss of compliance and increased stiffness of large conduit arteries, e.g. the aorta and its main branches. Large arterial stiffening means that the normal buffering capacity of large vessels is lost, such that blood pressure is abnormally high during systole. Loss of the normal elastic recoil means that blood pressure in the large arteries is abnormally low during diastole. Lowered diastolic blood pressure can reduce coronary blood flow, thereby exacerbating cardiac ischaemia in certain situations. High cardiac after-load causes hypertrophy of the cardiac muscle, which further increases myocardial oxygen demand and increases the risk of clinical or subclinical cardiac ischaemia. Left ventricular hypertrophy is likely to exacerbate angina in patients with pre-existing coronary atherosclerosis. In patients with low arterial compliance, the consequent increase in pulse pressure increases shear stress thereby exacerbating endothelial vascular damage caused by co-existent diabetes and lipid disorders. Narrowing and sclerosis of end-arterioles in the brain leads to lacunar and micro-infarcts and is probably a major contributor to dementia. The same process in the kidney leads to nephrosclerosis and loss of renal mass.

> *"In a very small number of patients there appears to be a particularly strong genetic basis for the development of hypertension"*

> *"Cardiac and vascular responses to high blood pressure result in functional and structural alterations that can sustain high blood pressure levels"*

Initial assessment in hypertension

Clinical history taking and physical examination should focus on determining:

- causes of hypertension
- contributory factors
- complications of hypertension
- cardiovascular disease risk factors (risk assessment)
- contraindications to specific drugs.

It is particularly important to determine any clinical history of established cardiovascular disease or diabetes mellitus, and to document any family history of hypertension or manifestations such as stroke or CAD affecting young family members. This should also include assessment of smoking status.

> *"High cardiac after-load causes hypertrophy of the cardiac muscle, which further increases myocardial oxygen demand"*

95

66 *It is particularly important to determine any clinical history of established cardiovascular disease or diabetes mellitus* 99

There are a number of simple investigations that should be used to assess all patients with newly diagnosed hypertension:

- dipstick urinalysis
- serum creatinine and electrolytes
- blood glucose
- lipid profile
- electrocardiogram (ECG).

One of the purposes of these routine investigations is to determine the extent of any target organ damage, for example proteinuria or haematuria as a crude marker of hypertensive nephropathy, or left ventricular hypertrophy as an indicator of increased cardiovascular risk. A further reason underlying basic routine laboratory assessment in all patients is to inform overall cardiovascular risk assessment, and the measurement of total:HDL cholesterol ratio is particularly important for predicting future risk.

66 *A further reason underlying basic routine laboratory assessment in all patients is to inform overall cardiovascular risk assessment* 99

Other investigations should not be performed routinely, but may be indicated in special situations. Specific investigations may be indicated for those with features suggesting secondary causes of isolated hypertension, for example phaeochromocytoma (Figure 56). Screening patients for phaeochromocytoma is usually by assessment of 24-hour urinary metanephrines or plasma metanephrine concentrations, whereas urinary vanillylmandelic acid (VMA) is inadequate due to a false negative rate in as many as 50% of patients. A thyroid-stimulating hormone (TSH) level is recommended only in patients with features suggestive of hyper-thyroidism. The resting ECG can be useful for determining left ventricular hypertrophy, but is less sensitive than echocardiography. Echocardiography is normally reserved for situations where there is difficulty determining whether to initiate therapy, or if indicated by other clinical findings such as arrhythmia or valvular cardiac problems.

Treatment of hypertension

66 *Specific investigations may be indicated for those with features suggesting secondary causes of isolated hypertension* 99

Every patient with hypertension requires assessment of global cardiovascular risk (see pages 21–29). The use of risk charts combining multiple independent cardiovascular risk factors in clinical practice has allowed better control of systolic blood pressure.[304] The overall level of risk should guide the intensity of treatment and follow-up and, therefore, the charts provide an overall indication of the need for medical intervention, rather than to determine only if blood pressure lowering treatment should be introduced.

General principles

The cardiovascular complications of hypertension are best treated with a combination of lifestyle modifications and pharmacological therapy.

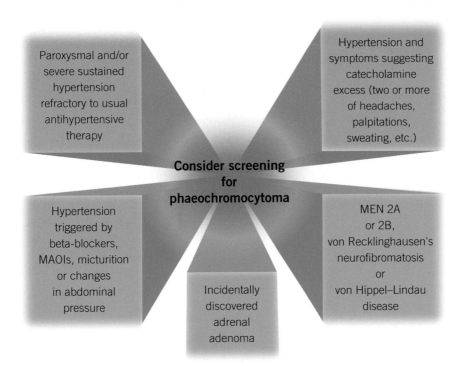

Fig. 56 Features suggesting underlying phaeochromocytoma that might prompt further screening investigations.

Hypertension trials have shown that treating hypertension leads predominantly to a reduction in stroke and, to a lesser extent, CAD and other cardiovascular event rates.[305,306] Meta-analyses of clinical trials in hypertension show that lowering systolic blood pressure by as little as 10–15 mmHg can reduce cardiovascular mortality by approximately one third over 5 years.[84] Further meta-analysis of placebo-controlled clinical trials has shown that antihypertensive treatment causes a 21% reduction in the risk of CAD compared with placebo.[307]

Treatment guidelines

Although clinical practice guidelines have become widespread in the medical literature, the impact that these have had on everyday clinical practice is uncertain. Key guidelines issuing advice on the detection, investigation and treatment of hypertension and its concomitant risk factors are provided by:

- European Joint Task Force of European and other Societies on Cardiovascular Disease Prevention in Clinical Practice
- WHO & International Society of Hypertension
- Joint National Committee on Prevention, Detection, Evaluation, and Treatment of High Blood Pressure.

Lowering systolic blood pressure by as little as 10–15 mmHg can reduce cardiovascular mortality by approximately one third over 5 years

> *The impact that clinical practice guidelines have had on everyday clinical practice is uncertain*

Guidelines produced by these societies are evidence-based and frequently updated to take account of new data from large clinical trials, and to incorporate the role of new treatments and other developments. They are designed to provide a framework for local and national societies to develop and implement their own local guidelines, within the context of specific regional needs. They take into account the need for global cardiovascular risk reduction and acknowledge the need to address hypertension treatment alongside cholesterol-lowering therapy, treatment for diabetes, smoking cessation and other lifestyle measures.

Landmark clinical trials that have informed the latest guidelines for antihypertensive treatment include large placebo-controlled trials in elderly patients. These have confirmed the benefits of treating hypertension in elderly patients with ISH. Other trials have provided more recent data that compare individual antihypertensive drugs, either as monotherapy or in combination regimens. A large body of evidence has clearly demonstrated lowering blood pressure in individuals with hypertension confers a significant reduction in cardio-vascular and CAD risk, and much recent attention has been focused on the ideal target blood pressure values. Many recent studies have attempted to address possible differences in efficacy between individual drug classes, including the ALLHAT, ANBP-2, INSIGHT, LIFE, STOP-2, and VALUE studies.[141,269,308–312] The antihypertensive treatment arm of the ASCOT study was the first large clinical trial to compare two different combination therapies in a high-risk group of patients with hypertension.[313]

> *Much recent attention has been focused on the ideal target blood pressure values*

Overall reductions of 5–6 mmHg in diastolic blood pressure (probably accompanied by an 8–10 mmHg reduction in systolic blood pressure) lead to a reduction in coronary endpoints by 15% and stroke by almost 40% over a 5-year period.[265,314] Meta-analyses of earlier trials have shown that all conventional "first-line" antihypertensive drugs offer similar long-term efficacy and overall safety. However recent clinical trial data have begun to identify the impact of specific adverse effect profiles when treatments are applied to large patient populations, for example an increased risk of heart failure associated with the use of doxazosin compared with diuretics,[141] ACE inhibitors or calcium channel blockers. Importantly, recent clinical trials have also identified important differences between antihypertensive classes with respect to cardiovascular outcome despite apparently similar blood pressure lowering effects, for example a lower incidence of diabetes mellitus in patients treated with losartan versus atenolol monotherapy, or a combination of perindopril and amlodipine versus a combination of atenolol and thiazide diuretic.[310,313]

> *All conventional 'first–line' antihypertensive drugs offer similar long–term efficacy and overall safety*

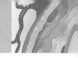

Clinical trial data: ISH

SHEP was a randomized placebo-controlled trial of chlortalidone in 4736 adults aged 60 years or above with ISH (systolic blood pressure >160 mmHg and diastolic blood pressure <90 mmHg).[247] The SHEP trial demonstrated that even a very modest reduction in systolic blood pressure caused a very significant reduction in fatal and non-fatal CAD and strokes, in addition to a near two-thirds reduction in the incidence of heart failure.[247]

The Syst-Eur study examined the effects of twice-daily nitrendipine (a dihydropyridine calcium channel blocker) in a placebo-controlled trial involving 4695 patients aged 60 years or older who had ISH (systolic blood pressure >160 mmHg and diastolic blood pressure <95 mmHg).[83] Active treatment led to a substantial reduction in the incidence of fatal and non-fatal cardiovascular endpoints.[83] The study involved a large cohort of patients with diabetes, and the rate of cardiovascular complications was significantly reduced in this subgroup too.[204]

There were remarkable similarities between the outcomes of the SHEP and Syst-Eur studies (Figure 57). A meta-analysis of trials in older patients with ISH, including data from the SHEP and Syst-Eur studies, found that a 10 mmHg reduction in systolic blood pressure sustained over 4 years led to an 18% decrease in cardiovascular mortality, a 26% reduction of all cardiovascular complications, a reduced incidence of stroke by 30%, and a 23% reduction in coronary events.

Clinical trial data: comparison between drug groups

ALLHAT study

One of the largest clinical trials on the treatment of hypertension is ALLHAT.[141,269] It was sponsored by the National Heart, Lung, and Blood Institute (NHBLI) in the USA, and recruited more than 42,000 study subjects worldwide. It involved a lipid-lowering arm and a blood pressure lowering arm, and the antihypertensive study was designed to compare the effects of thiazides (as a comparator group), ACE inhibitors, calcium channel blockers and alpha-blockers on the incidence of cardiovascular disease in a high-risk group of patients with hypertension.

The safety monitoring board terminated the alpha-blocker arm of the study prematurely because of an apparent increase in the incidence of heart failure in this group; this was a tertiary outcome measure of the study, and overall mortality was similar to that for other study groups. The study was completed for patients receiving drugs other than alpha-blockers; key findings included:

- all types of antihypertensive drugs significantly reduced systolic blood pressure; chlortalidone > amlodipine > lisinopril

❝Recent clinical trials have also identified important differences between antihypertensive classes with respect to cardiovascular outcome despite apparently similar blood pressure lowering effects ❞

❝The SHEP trial demonstrated that even a very modest reduction in systolic blood pressure caused a very significant reduction in fatal and non–fatal CAD and strokes ❞

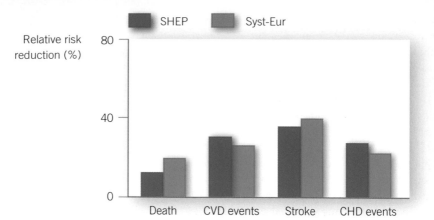

Fig. 57 Relative risk reduction in death and major cardiovascular outcomes in the SHEP and Syst-Eur studies.[83,247] CVD = cardiovascular disease; CHD = coronary heart disease.

- there were no differences between groups for primary outcome (combined fatal CAD or non-fatal MI); chlortalidone 11.5% vs amlodipine 11.3% vs lisinopril 11.4%
- there were no differences between the groups assigned to chlortalidone and calcium channel blocker for all six pre-specified secondary outcomes (all-cause mortality, combined coronary heart disease, stroke, combined cardiovascular disease, ESRD, and cancer or hospitalization for GI bleeding)
- there were no differences between the groups assigned to chlortalidone and ACE inhibitor for four out of six pre-specified secondary outcomes (all-cause mortality, combined coronary heart disease, ESRD, and cancer or hospitalization for GI bleeding). For the two other secondary outcomes, the lisinopril group had 15% higher risk of stroke, and 10% higher risk of combined cardiovascular disease, which included higher risks of CHD, hospitalized or fatal congestive heart failure, hospitalized or treated angina, and need for coronary revascularization
- in the assessment of components of secondary outcomes, the chlortalidone group had a lower incidence of congestive heart failure compared with the groups assigned to ACE inhibitor and calcium channel blocker.

The ALLHAT researchers concluded that thiazide-type diuretics should be considered as first-line pharmacological therapy in patients with hypertension, and that none of the comparatively newer antihypertensive drugs offered any significant overall benefit as initial therapy.

ANBP-2

The recently reported ANBP-2 study also found that the extent of blood pressure lowering and the risk of the primary endpoint (any cardiovascular event or death from any cause) were similar between the group receiving ACE-inhibitor therapy and those receiving diuretic therapy.[308] The ANBP-2 study compared outcomes with ACE inhibitors versus diuretics in more than 6000 elderly patients with hypertension (65–84 years old). Despite similar reductions in blood pressure, cardiovascular events and deaths from any cause showed greater reductions in those receiving ACE inhibitors compared with those receiving diuretic treatment, particularly in men.

INSIGHT

The INSIGHT trial recruited 6321 patients with hypertension and at least one additional cardiovascular risk factor to receive either nifedipine or a combination of hydrochlorothiazide and amiloride.[309] Blood pressure lowering and risk of the primary outcome (a combined endpoint of cardiovascular death, MI, heart failure, or stroke) were similar between the two groups, indicating that calcium channel blocker or diuretic-based therapy were equally efficacious.

LIFE

The LIFE study examined the effects of the AIIRA losartan versus the beta-blocker atenolol on cardiovascular endpoints in 9000 high-risk hypertensive patients (systolic blood pressure 160–200 mmHg or diastolic blood pressure 95–115 mmHg) with left ventricular hypertrophy. Although both were equally effective in achieving blood pressure lowering, losartan was superior in reducing cardiovascular morbidity and mortality, particularly among patients with diabetes. In particular, treatment with losartan appeared more effective in reducing the incidence of stroke, arrhythmia and new-onset diabetes (Figure 58).[310,315]

STOP-Hypertension

The STOP-Hypertension trial compared the effects of "old drug therapy" and "new drug therapy" in 6614 patients aged 70 years or older with severe hypertension. They were assigned to receive either beta-blockers or thiazide diuretics (group 1), an ACE inhibitor (group 2), or a calcium channel blocker (group 3). There were no significant differences in cardiovascular outcomes between the treatment groups, even when data from the ACE inhibitor and calcium channel blocker cohorts were pooled together, suggesting that a beta-blocker or thiazide-based regimen was as effective as calcium channel blocker or ACE inhibitor-based treatment in older patients.[311]

VALUE

The VALUE trial was designed to compare antihypertensive therapy using valsartan or amlodipine in a high-risk group of 15,245 patients

> *The ALLHAT researchers concluded that thiazide-type diuretics should be considered as first-line pharmacological therapy in patients with hypertension*

> *Cardiovascular events and deaths from any cause showed greater reductions in those receiving ACE inhibitors compared with those receiving diuretic treatment*

> *Blood pressure lowering and risk of the primary outcome were similar between the two groups, indicating that calcium channel blocker or diuretic-based therapy were equally efficacious*

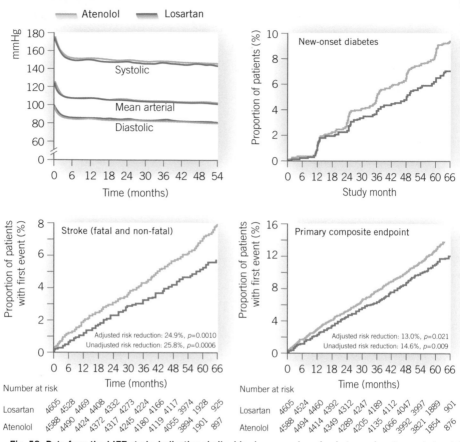

Fig. 58 Data from the LIFE study, indicating similar blood pressure lowering between losartan and atenolol, whereas losartan treatment was associated with a significantly lower incidence of cardiovascular disease, stroke and new-onset diabetes.[310,315] Reproduced with permission from Dahlof B, Devereux RB, Kjeldsen SE, et al. Cardiovascular morbidity and mortality in the Losartan Intervention For Endpoint reduction in hypertension study (LIFE): a randomised trial against atenolol. Lancet 2002;359:995–1003. ©Elsevier. and Lindholm LH, Ibsen H, Borch-Johnsen K, et al. Risk of new-onset diabetes in the Losartan Intervention For Endpoint reduction in hypertension study. J Hypertens 2002;20:1879–1886. ©Lippincott Williams and Wilkins.

with hypertension aged 50 years or older. Patients were followed up for a mean of 4.2 years. The study found that blood pressure lowering was more effective, especially at the start of the study, than with valsartan. The primary composite cardiovascular disease endpoint occurred in similar proportions of each group: 10.6% in the valsartan group and 10.4% in the amlodipine group (Figure 59).[312] The trend towards a more favourable outcome (reduced incidence of MI) with calcium channel blocker therapy versus AIIRA therapy might be explained, at least in part, by more effective blood pressure control (Figure 60). When the possible confounding effects of blood pressure differences

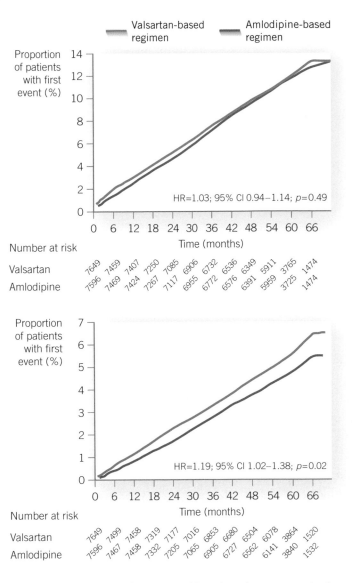

Fig. 59 Primary outcome measure in the VALUE study, which was similar in patients receiving either valsartan or amlodipine (top). Acute MI, a secondary outcome measure, was less frequent in the amlodipine treated group (bottom).

Reproduced with permission from Julius S, Kjeldsen S, Weber M, et al. Outcomes in hypertensive patients at high cardiovascular risk treated with regimens based on valsartan or amlodipine: the VALUE randomised trial. Lancet 2004;363:2022–2031. ©Elsevier.

❝The trend towards a more favourable outcome with calcium channel blocker therapy versus AIIRA therapy might be explained, at least in part, by more effective blood pressure control❞

were considered, by serial mean matching, then the outcomes in the two groups were very similar (Figure 61).[316]

ASCOT

The ASCOT study involved both a lipid-lowering therapy arm and antihypertensive study arm. The blood pressure lowering component of the ASCOT study was designed to compare a beta-blocker and thiazide-based regimen versus a calcium channel blocker and ACE

Fig. 60 Blood pressure differences between groups receiving either valsartan or amlodipine in the VALUE study. Reproduced with permission from Julius S, Kjeldsen S, Weber M, et al. Outcomes in hypertensive patients at high cardiovascular risk treated with regimens based on valsartan or amlodipine: the VALUE randomised trial. Lancet 2004;363:2022–2031. ©Elsevier

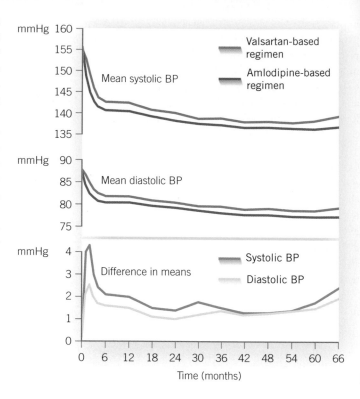

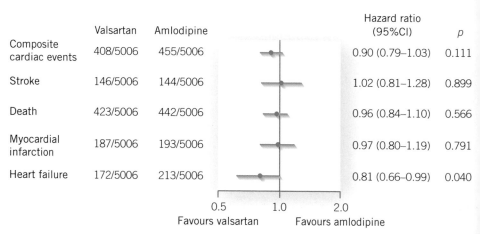

	Valsartan	Amlodipine		Hazard ratio (95%CI)	p
Composite cardiac events	408/5006	455/5006		0.90 (0.79–1.03)	0.111
Stroke	146/5006	144/5006		1.02 (0.81–1.28)	0.899
Death	423/5006	442/5006		0.96 (0.84–1.10)	0.566
Myocardial infarction	187/5006	193/5006		0.97 (0.80–1.19)	0.791
Heart failure	172/5006	213/5006		0.81 (0.66–0.99)	0.040

0.5   1.0   2.0

Favours valsartan   Favours amlodipine

Fig. 61 Outcomes of patients recruited to the VALUE study after serial median exact matching for blood pressure, gender, age and the presence or absence of coronary disease.[316] Reproduced with permission from Weber MA, Julius S, Kjeldsen SE, et al. Blood pressure dependent and independent effects of antihypertensive treatment on clinical events in the VALUE Trial. Lancet 2004;363:2049–2051. ©Elsevier

inhibitor-based regimen and involved treating 19,257 high-risk patients with hypertension.[313] The investigators reported similar blood pressure lowering in both groups (Figure 62), and a similar incidence in the composite primary cardiovascular endpoint of the study (Figure 63).[313] However the incidence of fatal and non-fatal stroke (Figure 64) and the incidence of new-onset diabetes (Figure 65) were significantly lower in the calcium channel blocker and ACE inhibitor group compared with those receiving beta-blocker and thiazide therapy.[313]

Conclusions

As more and more information has become available from large clinical trials, such as HOT,[202] the importance of escalating therapy towards progressively lower blood pressure targets has emerged. As a result, an increasing proportion of patients require combination therapy, often with three or more different antihypertensive drugs to attain target blood pressure. The need for concomitant antihypertensive therapy has confounded studies designed to compare one class of drugs with another, and led to some difficulty in interpreting findings. The recently reported ASCOT study is the first large clinical

❝The incidence of new–onset diabetes was significantly lower in the calcium channel blocker and ACE inhibitor group compared with those receiving beta–blocker and thiazide therapy❞

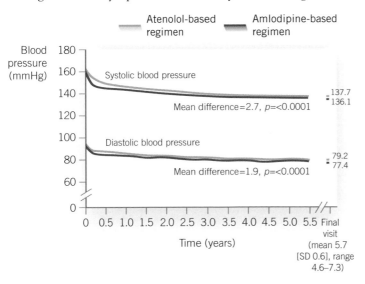

Fig. 62 Blood pressure lowering associated with beta-blocker +/- thiazide treatment versus calcium channel blocker +/- ACE inhibitor in the ASCOT study.

Reproduced with permission from Dahlof B, Sever PS, Poulter NR, et al. Prevention of cardiovascular events with an antihypertensive regimen of amlodipine adding perindopril as required versus atenolol adding bendroflumethiazide as required, in the Anglo-Scandinavian Cardiac Outcomes Trial-Blood Pressure Lowering Arm (ASCOT-BPLA): a multicentre randomised controlled trial. Lancet 2005;366:895–906. ©Elsevier

Fig. 63 Primary composite cardiovascular endpoint was similar in patients with hypertension who received beta-blocker +/- thiazide treatment or calcium channel blocker +/- ACE inhibitor treatment in the ASCOT study. Reproduced with permission from Dahlof B, Sever PS, Poulter NR, et al. Prevention of cardiovascular events with an antihypertensive regimen of amlodipine adding perindopril as required versus atenolol adding bendroflumethiazide as required, in the Anglo-Scandinavian Cardiac Outcomes Trial-Blood Pressure Lowering Arm (ASCOT-BPLA): a multicentre randomised controlled trial. Lancet 2005;366:895–906. ©Elsevier

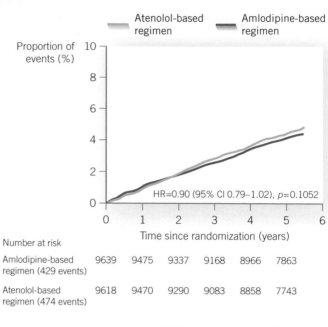

Fig. 64 Incidence of fatal and non-fatal stroke was significantly lower in patients with hypertension who received calcium channel blocker +/- ACE inhibitor treatment versus beta-blocker +/- thiazide treatment in the ASCOT study. Reproduced with permission from Dahlof B, Sever PS, Poulter NR, et al. Prevention of cardiovascular events with an antihypertensive regimen of amlodipine adding perindopril as required versus atenolol adding bendroflumethiazide as required, in the Anglo-Scandinavian Cardiac Outcomes Trial-Blood Pressure Lowering Arm (ASCOT-BPLA): a multicentre randomised controlled trial. Lancet 2005;366:895–906. ©Elsevier

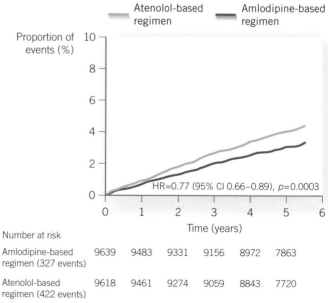

antihypertensive trial to compare two types of combination therapy: calcium channel blocker +/- ACE inhibitor versus beta-blocker +/- thiazide-type diuretic. There were striking similarities between the ASCOT and LIFE studies, suggesting that blockade of the renin-

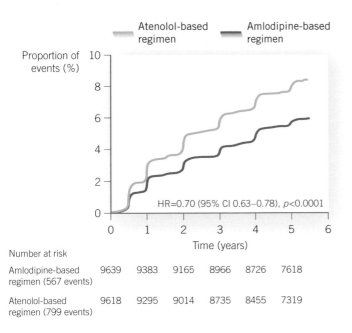

Proportion of events (%)

Atenolol-based regimen
Amlodipine-based regimen

HR=0.70 (95% CI 0.63–0.78), p<0.0001

Time (years)

Number at risk

Amlodipine-based regimen (567 events)	9639	9383	9165	8966	8726	7618
Atenolol-based regimen (799 events)	9618	9295	9014	8735	8455	7319

Fig. 65 Incidence of new-onset diabetes was significantly lower in patients with hypertension who received calcium channel blocker +/- ACE inhibitor treatment versus beta-blocker +/- thiazide treatment in the ASCOT study. Reproduced with permission from Dahlof B, Sever PS, Poulter NR, et al. Prevention of cardiovascular events with an antihypertensive regimen of amlodipine adding perindopril as required versus atenolol adding bendroflumethiazide as required, in the Anglo-Scandinavian Cardiac Outcomes Trial-Blood Pressure Lowering Arm (ASCOT-BPLA): a multicentre randomised controlled trial. Lancet 2005;366:895–906. ©Elsevier

angiotensin system, by AIIRA therapy or ACE inhibitors, might confer benefits that are over and above those anticipated from blood pressure lowering alone.

The HOPE trial assessed the role of an ACE inhibitor (ramipril) in preventing cardiovascular events in 9297 high-risk patients (55 years or older) who had evidence of vascular disease or diabetes or one other cardiovascular risk factor (hypertension, elevated total cholesterol levels, low HDL lipoprotein levels, cigarette smoking, or documented microalbuminuria). Ramipril was found to significantly reduce the rates of death, MI, and stroke compared with placebo.[317]

The EUROPA study provided further confirmation that ACE inhibitors may indeed have benefits beyond blood pressure reduction.[318] In this study perindopril demonstrated a 20% reduction in cardiovascular death, MI and cardiac arrest compared with placebo in over 12,000 patients with stable CAD but no evidence of heart failure or notable hypertension, i.e. at lower risk than the subjects in the HOPE study (Figure 66).

66The EUROPA study provided further confirmation that ACE inhibitors may indeed have benefits beyond blood pressure reduction 99

Pharmacological treatment

Initial therapy in most cases should be with an ACE inhibitor, in the absence of any contraindications. In elderly patients, or those of Afro-Caribbean origin, a low-dose thiazide diuretic or long-acting dihydropyridine calcium channel blocker would be expected to be

Fig. 66 Results of the EUROPA study. CV = cardiovascular. Reproduced with permission from the EUROPA Investigators. Efficacy of perindopril in reduction of cardiovascular events among patients with stable coronary artery disease: randomised, double-blind, placebo-controlled, multicentre trial (the EUROPA study). Lancet 2003;362:782–788. ©Elsevier

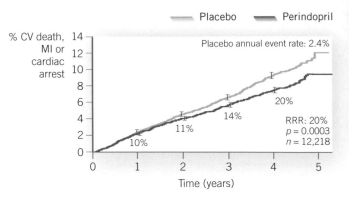

more effective and should be used as initial therapy. Note that short-acting calcium channel blockers are associated with an increased incidence of cardiovascular events and do not have a role in the treatment of hypertension.[319] The choice between diuretics and long-acting dihydropyridine calcium channel blockers is largely related to individual patient factors and economic constraints. However, preliminary evidence suggests that:

- diuretics are superior in preventing cardiac complications
- calcium channel blockers are superior in preventing cerebrovascular complications.[320,321]

66 Short-acting calcium channel blockers are associated with an increased incidence of cardiovascular events and do not have a role in the treatment of hypertension 99

Thiazide-like diuretics

Diuretics mainly have metabolic complications, although precipitation of gout and sexual dysfunction (2% over placebo) can occur.[322,323] Diuretic adverse effects are dose related, unusual at low doses and common at high doses.[324–326] Most of the blood pressure lowering effect occurs at diuretic doses equivalent to hydrochlorothiazide 25 mg/day or bendroflumethiazide 2.5 mg/day. High doses should be reserved for patients with resistant hypertension who have a demonstrated reduction in blood pressure as the dose is increased (reflecting a volume-dependent form of hypertension).

66 Using low doses of thiazide-like diuretics results in a low incidence of hypokalaemia 99

Rare or serious adverse effects including pancreatitis, rash, blood dyscrasia and renal cell carcinoma have been associated with thiazide-like diuretics. A retrospective analysis of data from the SHEP trial found that cardiovascular events were not prevented by chlortalidone if the baseline serum potassium was low (Figure 67).[327] Using low doses of thiazide-like diuretics (e.g. bendroflumethiazide 2.5 mg/day) results in a low incidence of hypokalaemia, which can be prevented by combination with a potassium-sparing diuretic (e.g. spironolactone) or an ACE inhibitor or AIIRA.

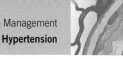

	Active treatment with chlortalidone		Placebo
	>3.5	<3.5	>3.5
Potassium (mmol/L)	>3.5	<3.5	>3.5
CVD event rate/1000 years	27.9	50	41.2
Systolic blood pressure (mmHg)	143±16	140±13	157±17

Long-acting dihydropyridine calcium channel blockers

The adverse effects of long-acting dihydropyridine calcium channel blockers are dose related, uncommon at low doses and common at high doses.[328–330] Adverse effects that commonly occur include ankle oedema, flushing and fatigue.[329] Unlike diuretics, calcium channel blockers have a relatively steep dose–response curve with greater blood pressure lowering effects gained by using higher doses.[329,330] Nevertheless, to minimize adverse effects, treatment is initiated at low doses and only titrated towards higher doses if tolerated.

Beta-blockers

Beta-blockers are relatively ineffective at reducing systolic blood pressure and, more importantly, are less effective than diuretics at preventing cardiovascular events in elderly hypertensive patients.[322,331] Beta-blockers are strongly indicated for secondary prevention of cardiovascular events in patients who have sustained a previous MI, and are regarded as highly effective in reducing mortality in patients at high risk of tachyarrhythmia.

The LIFE and ASCOT studies raised concerns that beta-blocker treatment might increase the risk of developing diabetes.[310,313] On the contrary, it is also possible that ACE inhibitor or AIIRA treatment might simply be more effective than other antihypertensive drug classes in preventing new-onset diabetes, and a deleterious effect of beta-blockers remains unproven at present. However, a comparison of two beta-blockers, metoprolol and carvedilol, in patients with hypertension and diabetes demonstrated better glycaemic control with the third-generation beta-blocker carvedilol compared with the second-generation metoprolol.[332] The randomized, double-blind, parallel-group GEMINI trial included 1235 patients already receiving an ACE inhibitor or AIIRA and revealed an increase in HbA_{1c} in patients receiving metoprolol (+0.15%, p<0.001) but not those receiving carvedilol (+0.02%, p=0.65). Insulin resistance also improved with carvedilol but not metoprolol and progression to micro-

Fig. 67 Changes in cardiovascular disease outcome measures in the SHEP study during treatment with chlortalidone, in patients with and without hypokalaemia.[327] CVD = cardiovascular disease.

"Beta–blockers are strongly indicated for secondary prevention of cardiovascular events in patients who have sustained a previous MI"

109

albuminuria was less frequent with carvedilol than metoprolol. This study suggests that there may be differences between beta-blockers regarding their metabolic effects, possibly due to differences in receptor-binding profiles (third-generation beta-blockers also block alpha$_1$-receptors), although further studies are required to establish if these differences translate into improved cardiovascular outcomes.

Alpha-blockers

66 Co-existent hypertension and benign prostatic hyperplasia requiring treatment is a special situation where alpha-blockers might be indicated as monotherapy 99

Alpha-blockers are less effective in preventing cardiovascular events than diuretics and, due to the apparently increased risk of congestive heart failure, are not recommended as monotherapy. Co-existent hypertension and benign prostatic hyperplasia requiring treatment is a special situation where alpha-blockers might be indicated as monotherapy. However, they are generally introduced only as third-line agents, or where other treatments have not been tolerated or effective.

ACE inhibitors and AIIRAs

66 AIIRAs are generally reserved for patients in whom ACE inhibitor therapy is not tolerated due to cough 99

The safety and efficacy of both ACE inhibitor and AIIRA therapy in hypertension have now been established in large-scale clinical trials. There is little evidence of benefit associated with any particular ACE inhibitor within this class of drugs although in order to obtain sustained blood pressure reduction those with short duration are best avoided, for example captopril or enalapril. Those with a longer duration of action, for example lisinopril or perindopril, might be expected to give more sustained blood pressure lowering over a full 24-hour period, minimizing the need for frequent dosing and the risk of adverse effects. A large body of clinical trial data supports the use of losartan in the treatment of hypertension but, predominantly for economic reasons, AIIRAs are generally reserved for patients in whom ACE inhibitor therapy is not tolerated due to cough. There is no evidence of any clinically relevant difference in outcomes associated with AIIRA versus ACE inhibitor therapy in patients with hypertension.

Combining or switching drugs

66 Most of the blood pressure lowering effects of antihypertensive drugs are achieved at a moderate dose 99

To maximize the effectiveness of antihypertensive therapy, treatments often need to be combined or switched to more effective alternatives. The maximum reduction of systolic blood pressure expected from any single drug treatment is around 10 mmHg. Most of the blood pressure lowering effects of antihypertensive drugs are achieved at a moderate dose, while common adverse effects tend to occur at higher doses. Therefore, adding agents at moderate doses is generally recommended if there is a failure to achieve the blood pressure target with a single drug, rather than simply escalating the dose of any single agent. A simple system for combining antihypertensive agents, known as the ABCD system, is recommended by the BHS and illustrated in Figure 68.[333] It is generally considered that the combination of a beta-blocker and a thiazide diuretic is associated with a higher incidence of diabetes than other combinations, particularly in older patients. Thus the preferred triple therapy is ACE inhibitor + calcium channel blocker + thiazide diuretic, with beta-blockers reserved for those with a specific indication, e.g. CAD.

Switching between first-line drugs can be an effective way to reduce blood pressure, but a higher number of switches in therapy has been associated with a higher rate of discontinuing medications.[334,335] Even with multiple drug switches, many patients with mild-to-moderate hypertension (systolic blood pressure 140–160 mmHg) will not achieve current blood pressure targets and combination therapy will be required.[334]

> *The combination of a beta-blocker and a thiazide diuretic is associated with a higher incidence of diabetes than other combinations, particularly in older patients*

Very elderly patients

There is little information from randomized controlled trials on the treatment of very elderly patients, e.g. >80 years. A recent meta-analysis provides some evidence that blood pressure lowering reduces stroke incidence by one-third, and heart failure by 40%, but this was associated with a non-significant trend towards higher mortality overall.[336] Therefore the decision to initiate therapy in patients over 80

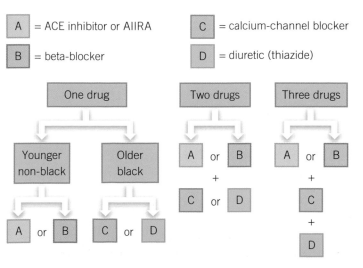

Fig. 68 **The ABCD system for choosing antihypertensive therapy.**[333] Reproduced with permission from Schachter M, Monkman D. Hypertension. Oxford: Elsevier, 2004. ©Elsevier

years of age needs to consider the overall health status of the patient and the risks of hypertension and cardiovascular disease relative to other competing causes of morbidity and death.

Postural hypotension

Some of the key factors predisposing to postural hypotension are:

- co-morbidity (e.g. diabetes)
- drug treatment in the very elderly
- intermittent compliance.

66 In some older individuals postural hypotension occurs only after being upright for more than 30 minutes 99

Monitoring for this symptom should occur before and during therapy, and symptomatic patients may require reversal of therapy targets. Postural hypotension is common in elderly patients regardless of hypertension, and a drop in systolic blood pressure of 20 mmHg occurs in 15% of those aged 65–74 years and in 20% of those aged over 75 years. The significance is that drug therapy can exaggerate this effect and increase the incidence of symptomatic hypotension. In some older individuals postural hypotension occurs only after being upright for more than 30 minutes or after meals. Treatment should be initiated at low doses and titrated gradually. This is especially important for antihypertensive drugs associated with a high incidence of postural hypotension (e.g. ACE inhibitors and alpha-blockers).

Need for specialist intervention

Most hypertensive patients are best managed in primary care. Practices with multidisciplinary team support are particularly well adapted. Referral to a medical specialist or a hypertension specialist occurs for a variety of reasons depending on the experience, expertise and comfort level of the family physician as well as the complexity and difficulty of the patient's issues.

66 If treatment targets cannot be obtained with a drug regimen the practitioner feels comfortable prescribing, referral should be considered 99

Hypertensive urgencies and emergencies are optimally cared for in specialized centres.

If a secondary cause of hypertension that requires specialty intervention is suspected on diagnostic testing, a referral is appropriate. Screening and initial diagnostic testing for the common causes of secondary hypertension are available to many urban family physicians. However, in some centres obtaining 24-hour ABPM or some specialized tests requires referral.

Secondary hypertension is more common in those with:

- abnormal screening tests
- severe or drug-resistant hypertension
- rapid changes in blood pressure.

Referral should be considered for these patients.

Also in general, if treatment targets cannot be obtained with a drug regimen the practitioner feels comfortable prescribing, referral should be considered.

In some cases, a referral to reinforce the importance of hypertension and its treatment and goals of treatment is reasonable.

Importance of hypertension as a cardiovascular risk factor in diabetes

Patients with diabetes and hypertension have a high risk for cardiovascular events: 20–30% over 10 years.[337] Renal function declines faster in patients with diabetes if they have co-existent hypertension.[233,338] Treatment of hypertension would be expected to confer at least as much benefit, and possibly greater cardiovascular risk reduction, in patients with diabetes compared with age-matched hypertensive patients without diabetes.[339–341] Indirect comparisons in trials such as the UKPDS suggest that the benefits of aggressive blood pressure lowering may even exceed those from aggressive glycaemic control. It must be recognized, however, that the UKPDS investigators were far more successful at improving blood pressure than they were at improving HbA_{1c} (only a 0.9% difference between the intensive and conventional policy groups). More strict blood pressure control (average 144/82 mmHg) compared with less tight control (average 154/87 mmHg) led to an overall mortality reduction of 32% in patients with diabetes.[341]

> **"In diabetes the benefits of aggressive blood pressure lowering may even exceed those from aggressive glycaemic control"**

Epidemiology of hypertension in diabetes

Hypertension incidence increases by 3% for each year of diabetes and is three times more likely in patients with proteinuria and 23% more likely in those with higher HbA_{1c} levels.[90] Measurement of blood pressure is a simple method for screening patients with both type 1 and type 2 diabetes to identify those at particularly high risk for the development of nephropathy.

> **"Lifestyle measures are especially important to emphasize in patients with co-existent diabetes and hypertension"**

Management

In patients with diabetes, control of blood pressure and blood lipids to established targets would be expected to confer substantial benefits in

Clinic blood pressure (mmHg)		
	No diabetes	**Diabetes**
Optimal treated blood pressure	<140/85	<130/80
Audit standard	<150/90	<140/80

Fig. 69 Target blood pressure values in patients with treated hypertension with and without co-existent diabetes.[342]

this high-risk patient group. Current BHS target blood pressures are presented in Figure 69.[342]

Lifestyle measures are especially important to emphasize in patients with co-existent diabetes and hypertension (summarized in Figure 70). Implementation of these measures will reduce HbA_{1c} concentrations and improve glycaemic control and cause a modest reduction in blood pressure.

Blood pressure can be brought under control in people with diabetes with appropriate use of medication and persistence over time.[135,343]

Fig. 70 Lifestyle measures to enhance cardiovascular risk reduction in patients with co-existent diabetes mellitus and hypertension.

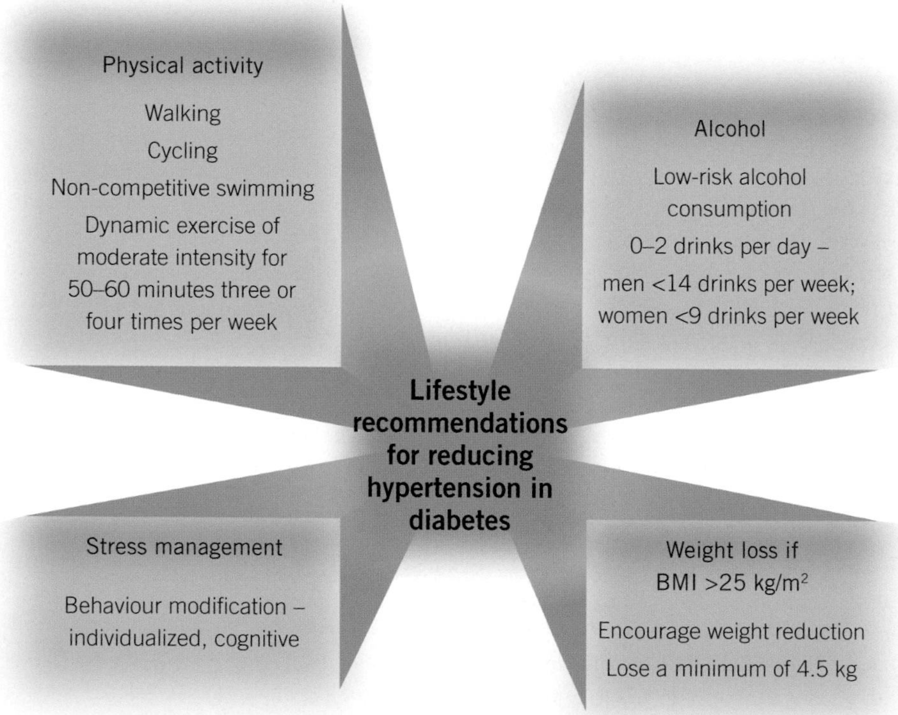

Target blood pressure values for people with diabetes are to attain:
- systolic blood pressure <130 mmHg
- diastolic blood pressure <80 mmHg.

Neither the UKPDS nor the HOT study demonstrated a threshold below which benefit did not occur. Because the effect size diminishes with lower achieved blood pressure and statistical benefit can only be demonstrated to 130/80 mmHg, blood pressure targets for

Physical activity

Walking
Cycling
Non-competitive swimming
Dynamic exercise of moderate intensity for 50–60 minutes three or four times per week

Alcohol

Low-risk alcohol consumption
0–2 drinks per day – men <14 drinks per week; women <9 drinks per week

Lifestyle recommendations for reducing hypertension in diabetes

Stress management

Behaviour modification – individualized, cognitive

Weight loss if BMI >25 kg/m²

Encourage weight reduction
Lose a minimum of 4.5 kg

diabetes have been set at this level. Large reductions in blood pressure lead to large reductions in the risk of events. Therefore the clinician may decide to aggressively decrease a higher blood pressure even though this usually requires multiple medications.

Although small reductions in blood pressure continue to lead to a reduction in risk, the proportionally smaller benefits accruing when blood pressure is nearing its target may lead the clinician to be more conservative when considering adding more medications at this point.

When treating patients with renal insufficiency and a creatinine clearance <30 mL/min (0.25 mL/s) or a creatinine level >150 mmol/L, the choice of antihypertensive agent is the same except that a loop diuretic should be considered as a substitute for low-dose thiazide treatment. This affords better control of circulating volume and blood pressure. After initiation of ACE inhibitor or AIIRA therapy, serum creatinine and potassium levels should be measured at baseline, 1–2 weeks after initiation and after any substantial increase in dose. If the creatinine level increases by more than 30% or the potassium level exceeds the upper limit of the local laboratory's normal range, the dose of ACE inhibitor should be reviewed. A rise in creatinine of up to 30% results from a drop in intraglomerular pressures when compensatory increases in efferent arteriolar pressure are lost.

> *Neither the UKPDS nor the HOT study demonstrated a threshold below which benefit did not occur*

Hypertension in patients with renal disease

Renal disease is an emerging cardiovascular risk factor. Even subtle renal disease (microalbuminuria) indicates a substantially increased risk for cardiovascular events.[344] Therefore blood pressure targets are even more aggressive in patients with renal disease or with proteinuria >1 g protein/24 hours: target systolic blood pressures <130 mmHg and <125 mm Hg, respectively.[345]

> *Blood pressure targets are even more aggressive in patients with renal disease*

Hypertension in obese patients

Patients with obesity tend to have reduced insulin sensitivity, which can be impaired further by diuretics and beta-blockers. The clinical significance of this finding is not entirely clear, but suggests that these may be less preferred to other antihypertensive drugs in obese patients, for example, calcium channel blockers, which appear to have few effects on insulin sensitivity. Given that activation of the renin-angiotensin-aldosterone system is thought to contribute to hypertension in obese patients, ACE inhibitors and AIIRAs would appear to be a logical first-line therapy for hypertension in patients with obesity, and further work is required to examine the effect of different therapies on clinical outcomes.

> *ACE inhibitors and AIIRAs would appear to be a logical first-line therapy for hypertension in patients with obesity*

> *The role of combination therapy has become established into treatment of the majority of patients with hypertension*

Conclusions

Hypertension is a major independent cardiovascular risk factor that is highly prevalent in Western societies, and becoming more so. Its impact on risk is even more striking in patients with other established risk factors, for example diabetes mellitus or hypercholesterolaemia. Optimum risk reduction requires clinical awareness and detection of hypertension, especially in high-risk populations, and a concerted effort should be made to achieve progressively decreasing blood pressure targets. The role of combination therapy has become established into treatment of the majority of patients with hypertension, and it is likely that this will be assisted by development of novel fixed-dose drug combinations in the future.

Antiplatelet therapy

The antithrombotic trialists' collaboration conducted a meta-analysis of randomized trials of antiplatelet therapy for the prevention of death, MI and stroke in high-risk patients concluding that antiplatelet therapy reduced the risk of serious vascular events by about 25%.[346] Furthermore in patients with established CAD there is a 37% proportional reduction in serious vascular events associated with antiplatelet therapy. Aspirin was well tolerated in the HOT study in which it reduced all cardiovascular events by 15% and all MI by 36% compared with placebo.[202] The absolute benefits of aspirin therapy are greatest in those with highest cardiovascular risk (Figure 71).[347] However the adverse effects of treatment are significant, including haemorrhage and peptic ulceration. Low-dose aspirin (75–100 mg) has

> *The absolute benefits of aspirin therapy are greatest in those with highest cardiovascular risk*

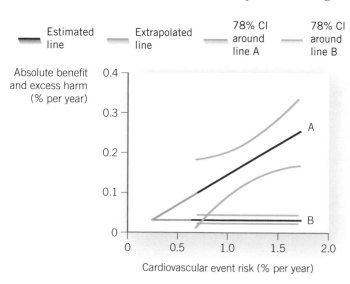

Fig. 71 The absolute benefit obtained from aspirin therapy (line A), alongside the absolute harm associated with aspirin therapy (line B). Reproduced with permission from Sanmuganathan PS, Ghahramani P, Jackson PR, et al. Aspirin for primary prevention of coronary heart disease: safety and absolute benefit related to coronary risk derived from meta-analysis of randomised trials. Heart 2001;85:265–271. ©BMJ Publishing Group

been shown to provide similar risk reduction to higher doses of aspirin while reducing the risk of gastrointestinal side-effects and is therefore recommended for daily use in the long-term prevention of serious vascular events in high-risk patients.[348]

In order that the beneficial effects of cardiovascular risk reduction prevail over potential adverse effects, it is recommended that aspirin be considered only for high-risk patients (>15% 10-year CAD risk). In patients with 10-year CAD risk between 10% and 15%, the absolute benefits of aspirin are not as great, reducing the risk/benefit ratio, such that in patients with 10-year CAD risk <10% the adverse risks of therapy are likely to outweigh potential benefits, making antiplatelet therapy inadvisable in this group (Figure 72).

Furthermore it is acknowledged that in patients with poorly controlled hypertension antiplatelet therapy poses an increased risk of intracranial haemorrhage.[349] In view of this, current guidelines advocate controlling blood pressure to target values before contemplating antiplatelet treatment in high-risk individuals.

In patients who are intolerant of aspirin an alternative antiplatelet agent should be considered. Clopidogrel is generally considered the first-line alternative agent and appears to be at least as effective as aspirin in preventing acute coronary events. The CAPRIE study in nearly 20,000 patients with atherosclerotic vascular disease demonstrated a greater reduction in risk of ischaemic stroke, MI or vascular death with clopidogrel (75 mg) compared with medium-dose (325 mg) aspirin (8.7% overall relative risk reduction in favour of clopidogrel, p=0.043).[350]

> *66In patients with poorly controlled hypertension antiplatelet therapy poses an increased risk of intracranial haemorrhage 99*

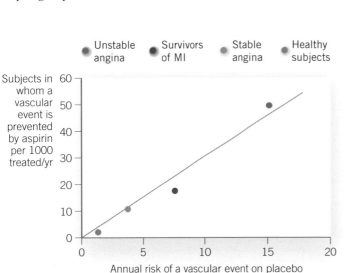

Fig. 72 Subjects in whom a vascular event is prevented by aspirin per 1000 treated/year versus annual risk of a vascular event on placebo. Reproduced with permission from Patrono C, Coller B, Dalen JE, et al. Platelet-Active Drugs: the relationship among dose, effectiveness, and side effects. Chest 1998;114:470S–488S. ©American College of Chest Physicians

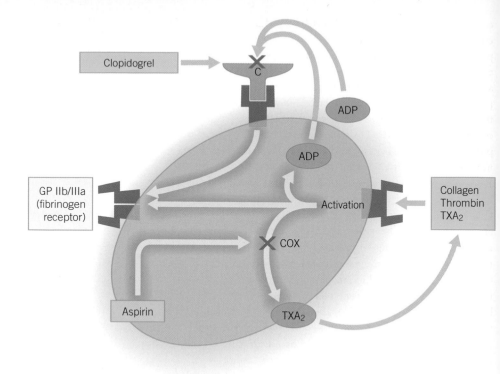

Fig. 73 Pathways resulting in platelet activation/aggregation. COX = cyclooxygenase; ADP = adenosine diphosphate; TXA_2 = thromboxane A_2; C = clopidogrel. Reproduced with permission from Katz R, Purcell H. Acute Coronary Syndromes. Oxford: Elsevier, 2006. ©Elsevier

Dual antiplatelet therapy

The modes of action for aspirin and clopidogrel are thought to be complementary (Figure 73) leading to investigation of using the two compounds in combination. Indeed the results of the CURE study have led to recommendations that clopidogrel is added to aspirin therapy for 1 year following acute coronary syndromes without ST-elevation (unstable angina and non-ST-segment elevation MI).[348] Over 12,500 patients were randomized to receive either clopidogrel or placebo in addition to aspirin for 3–12 months (mean 9 months) following a qualifying event and the primary outcome was a composite of death from cardiovascular causes, non-fatal MI or stroke.[351] A 20% relative risk reduction in the primary outcome was seen with clopidogrel in addition to aspirin compared with aspirin monotherapy (p<0.001). However, this was associated with an increased incidence of major bleeding, although there was no excess rate of fatal bleeding, bleeding requiring surgical intervention or haemorrhagic stroke.

The benefit of clopidogrel added to aspirin compared with aspirin monotherapy was investigated in over 15,000 patients at high cardiovascular risk in the CHARISMA trial.[352] Both patients with established atherosclerotic disease (CAD, cerebrovascular disease or peripheral artery disease) and high-risk asymptomatic patients were enrolled into this study to enable the role of combination clopidogrel and aspirin to be established in both secondary and high-risk primary prevention of atherothrombotic events. Preliminary results indicate that while there was no overall benefit of dual antiplatelet therapy compared with aspirin monotherapy in the primary endpoint, prevention of first MI, stroke or death from cardiovascular causes at 28 months (6.8% with dual therapy vs 7.3% with aspirin monotherapy, RR=0.93, 95% CI 0.83–1.05, p=0.22), there was a suggestion of benefit in patients with symptomatic atherothrombosis (documented CAD, documented cerebrovascular disease or documented peripheral arterial disease).[352] The symptomatic subgroup (n=12,153) experienced a significant reduction in the primary endpoint (6.9% with dual therapy vs 7.9% with aspirin monotherapy, RR = 0.88, 95% CI 0.77–0.998, p=0.046) with no significant increase in severe bleeding (1.6% vs 1.4%, p=0.39) although there was an increase in moderate bleeding (2.1% vs 1.3%, p<0.001). However, the asymptomatic group (those with multiple risk factors but no documented atherothrombotic disease) experienced no significant reduction in the primary endpoint, although the incidence of bleeding complications was increased. The authors conclude that dual antiplatelet therapy should not be used in the broad population tested; however, the benefits of dual antiplatelet therapy warrant further investigation in people with established vascular disease.

Dipyridamole is as effective as aspirin alone in preventing transient ischaemic attacks and stroke. The combination of aspirin and dipyridamole appears more effective than either drug given as monotherapy for stroke prevention, and should be considered for patients who have suffered a recurrent event despite treatment with either alone.[353] However, the addition of dipyridamole to aspirin has not been shown to produce additional reductions in other serious vascular events compared with aspirin alone and there is no strong basis for recommending this combination in patients with ischaemic heart disease.[348]

More comparative data are needed to establish the role of non-aspirin antiplatelet therapy, and to examine the potential benefits of various combination regimens. A number of ongoing studies are examining these issues, for example the PRoFESS study, which aims to compare combined aspirin and dipyridamole to clopidogrel monotherapy in more than 15,000 high-risk patients, expected to report in 2008.[354]

"The benefits of dual antiplatelet therapy warrant further investigation in people with established vascular disease"

"The combination of aspirin and dipyridamole appears more effective than either drug given as monotherapy for stroke prevention"

"More comparative data are needed to establish the role of non-aspirin antiplatelet therapy, and to examine the potential benefits of various combination regimens"

119

Patient issues and compliance

A variety of factors can suggest lack of adherence to therapy, for example:

- lack of response to appropriate therapy
- failure to attend follow-up visits
- patients indicating that they do not agree with therapy
- failure to fill prescriptions.[355]

The following question can be helpful during clinic visits: "many people have difficulty taking drugs, are you having any difficulties?" Non-adherence can in part be prevented by ensuring that patients are well informed about:

- their current level of cardiovascular risk
- benefits of therapy
- reasons for and the expected outcomes of the selected therapy.

Determining the cause of non-adherence may be critical to tailoring specific interventions. For example a patient who repeatedly forgets to take medications at home could be advised to keep a second supply at work or in the car. Non-specific interventions such as increasing the frequency of office visits, medication dispensers (i.e. dosette boxes) and self-monitoring of blood pressure or blood sugar may improve adherence to therapy.

Patients should be warned that they will probably need more than one medication to bring their blood pressure under control, and given education to enable them to cope with adhering to complex regimens involving multiple medications. A focus on the positive aspects of therapy will help to gain its acceptance. Statements that can reinforce a positive message include:

- "the average patient with diabetes requires three antihypertensive agents to bring blood pressure to target and some even more"
- "bringing your blood pressure towards the target blood pressure or below will greatly increase the number of days you will live without serious illnesses such as stroke, heart attack and kidney failure, and the effect is cumulative: the longer you are on medication, the greater the benefit."

In recognition of the increased demand for combination medications, as outlined above, the pharmaceutical industry has renewed its interest in developing fixed-dose combinations, a trend that promises to continue in the future.[356] Targets may not be achieved for many patients, even with multiple medications. However, it is often possible to achieve the target with persistence over a period of years. Compliance with treatment can be improved by integrating multiple risk reduction strategies.

Non-pharmacological recommendations should include strategies for improving adherence to medication prescriptions. Self-monitoring

A patient who repeatedly forgets to take medications at home could be advised to keep a second supply at work or in the car

The pharmaceutical industry has renewed its interest in developing fixed-dose combinations, a trend that promises to continue in the future

Patients should be reminded of the multiple potential benefits of lifestyle interventions

of blood glucose or blood pressure not only allows for appropriate titration of medication, it also provides important feedback on the immediate impact of lifestyle changes. The frequency of testing should be individualized. With increasing time there is often increasing reliance on medications to the detriment of lifestyle changes. Referral for "refresher" education sessions may be of value, and patients should be reminded of the multiple potential benefits of lifestyle interventions, for example that efforts to lose weight may achieve both blood pressure and lipid lowering in addition to improved glycaemic control.

❝Each form of therapy produces an independent reduction in relative risk ❞

Conclusion

A fundamental concept behind treatment of cardiovascular risk factors is that the benefit of therapy will be cumulative. This potential benefit is illustrated in Figure 74. Each form of therapy produces an independent reduction in relative risk. To estimate total risk reduction, relative risk reductions are multiplied such that two interventions providing a 30% risk reduction would provide approximately 50% relative risk reduction when combined $(1 - (0.7 \times 0.7))$. Simultaneous use of aspirin, a beta-blocker, a statin and an ACE inhibitor has been estimated to provide a 75% cumulative relative risk reduction based on the results of landmark trials.[357] Thus treatment of all major modifiable cardiovascular risk factors should reduce overall risk by over 75%.[24]

❝Ongoing research into new chemical entities is likely to produce more compounds treating multiple risk factors simultaneously ❞

The benefits of a healthy lifestyle should continually be reinforced. However, it is also important that once levels of cardiovascular risk begin to escalate the limitations of lifestyle intervention are recognized and appropriate pharmacological therapy is introduced in a timely fashion. Hypertension, dyslipidaemia, obesity and diabetes appear to have some common underlying pathogenetic components leading to some synergistic actions of their respective treatments. Treating the patient holistically considering their total cardiovascular risk can allow healthcare professionals to exploit this synergy. Indeed ongoing research into new chemical entities is likely to produce more compounds treating multiple risk factors simultaneously. In the future the idea of treating individual cardiovascular risk factors may become obsolete, and all patients will be treated according to an overall assessment of their cardiovascular risk.

Fig. 74 The relative risk reduction and cumulative relative risk associated with the presence of increasing numbers of interventions to reduce cardiovascular risk.[24]

Therapy	Relative risk reduction (%)	Cumulative RR
LDL lowering (statin)	−30	0.70
Aspirin	−25	0.52
Blood pressure control	−20	0.42
Fibrates/nicotinic acid	−20	0.34
Weight loss/exercise	−20	0.27

Case study 1

When to initiate antihypertensive therapy

A 29-year-old woman is referred to the Cardiovascular Risk Clinic for assessment. She has no significant past medical history of note and, until recently, had been taking the combined oral contraceptive pill (COCP) but no other regular medications. During a routine check-up at a reproductive health clinic 3 months ago, her blood pressure was found to be 138/104 mmHg. Her blood pressure was still high when rechecked by her GP, who recommended stopping the COCP and using a barrier method of contraception. Three weeks later, blood pressure averaged 128/102 mmHg, and she was referred to the clinic for further advice.

" The combined oral contraceptive pill might be expected to cause a very small increase in blood pressure "

Management issues

- In young women, the COCP might be expected to cause a very small increase in blood pressure in many patients. However a small proportion may experience a significant rise in blood pressure. This effect might persist for several weeks to months after discontinuing the COCP. Therefore, it is important to allow a sufficient observation period before concluding that blood pressure has failed to normalize after COCP discontinuation. The risk of blood pressure elevation is lower, but not negligible, for preparations that have a low or zero oestrogen component.

- Overall cardiovascular risk is low, based on the young age and female gender of the patient. While it is important to consider the potential contribution of other cardiovascular risk factors, for example cholesterol profile, smoking status, and family history, young patients can often be afforded a longer period of blood pressure monitoring prior to initiation of drug therapy. This will depend on the severity of the blood pressure elevation, presence of target organ damage, willingness of the patient to implement lifestyle modifications, and patient preference to delay embarking on potentially lifelong therapy.

" Young patients can often be afforded a longer period of blood pressure monitoring prior to initiation of drug therapy "

Follow-up

Further blood pressure recordings several months after discontinuing the COCP gave a consistently high diastolic reading of around 94–110 mmHg. The patient weighed 112 kg, representing a BMI of 38.1 kg/m², and stated that her weight had increased significantly over the past 2 years, after stopping smoking. There was no family history of hypertension or cardiovascular disease. A 24-hour ABPM showed mean daytime blood pressure of 112/84 mmHg. She was diagnosed with diastolic hypertension, on the basis of her persistently elevated clinic readings. During clinic, there was discussion of means by which she might modify her diet and incorporate regular aerobic exercise so as to promote weight loss. The patient was reluctant to take antihypertensive medication at this stage. It was agreed that she would make a determined effort to lose weight, and the issue of antihypertensive therapy would be revisited in 6 months.

66 The patient was reluctant to take antihypertensive medication at this stage 99

Case study 2

Significance of end-organ damage

A 55-year-old male heavy smoker, referred to the hypertension clinic by his GP, had been diagnosed with hypertension 3 years earlier. Initial blood pressure recordings were around 180/110 mmHg, which initially responded well to atenolol 100 mg daily, but this was subsequently withdrawn due to fatigue and muscle cramps. He had been taking modified-release nifedipine 60 mg daily and lisinopril 40 mg daily for many months. A 24-hour ambulatory blood pressure monitor indicated inadequate blood pressure control, and bendroflumethiazide 2.5 mg daily was added to his other treatments. Despite treatment escalation, his blood pressure remained elevated with clinic recordings that varied: 146–164/88–94 mmHg. Blood tests showed sodium 140 mmol/L, potassium 4.0 mmol/L, urea 9.8 mmol/L, and creatinine 224 µmol/L. Around 9 months earlier, urea was 6.4 mmol/L and creatinine 114 µmol/L, and in view of the rise in creatinine, his GP advised discontinuation of bendroflumethiazide and lisinopril, and arranged an urgent clinic appointment.

66 Despite treatment escalation, his blood pressure remained elevated with clinic recordings that varied: 146–164/88–94 mmHg 99

Management issues

- It can be difficult to distinguish renal impairment arising as a complication of severe hypertension or as an adverse effect of treatment, particularly after ACE inhibitors and AIIRAs.
- If renal impairment is a consequence of inadequately controlled hypertension then there may also be evidence of target organ damage elsewhere, for example retinopathy or left ventricular hypertrophy.

66 There may also be evidence of target organ damage elsewhere, for example retinopathy or left ventricular hypertrophy 99

- Blockade of the renin-angiotensin-aldosterone system may precipitate acute renal impairment in patients with renovascular insufficiency, which is most likely in elderly patients, and those with established vascular disease affecting other sites, for example CAD and peripheral vascular disease.
- Renovascular disease is significantly more prevalent in patients with diabetes, who have much to gain from treatment with ACE inhibitors or AIIRAs but who are also at greatest risk of developing renal impairment.
- A further possibility is that renal impairment might underlie hypertension, either due to significant renal artery stenosis or due to intrinsic renal pathology.
- In a relatively young patient, with blood pressure that is difficult to control, it is worth considering further renal investigations for possible underlying causes.

"Renovascular disease is significantly more prevalent in patients with diabetes"

Follow-up

Urinalysis of this patient showed trace haematuria and proteinuria. Fundi appeared normal, and resting ECG was normal. His previous medications were re-introduced, and magnetic resonance imaging of renal vasculature was performed: this did not identify any significant arterial insufficiency or any specific structural renal abnormality. Spironolactone was added to his previous medications, and at his most recent follow-up appointment, blood pressure was 144/84 mmHg and serum creatinine 128 μmol/L. In retrospect, it seems that renal impairment could not be explained solely by the combination of ACE inhibitor with his other medications, because he has subsequently been able to tolerate these. Other factors, for example dehydration or intercurrent illness, may also precipitate renal impairment in patients receiving ACE inhibitors or AIIRAs.

"Renal impairment could not be explained solely by the combination of ACE inhibitor with his other medications"

Case study 3

When to initiate cholesterol-lowering therapy?

A 57-year-old woman is referred to the Cardiology Outpatient Clinic for review. She had recently been assessed in the Acute Medical Admissions Unit with a short history of exertional chest pain, which had responded within several hours of treatment with sublingual nitrate, high-concentration oxygen, and oral atenolol administration. On discharge from hospital, she had been prescribed atenolol 50 mg daily, aspirin 75 mg daily, sublingual glyceryl trinitrate as required, and omeprazole 20 mg daily. On recounting her symptoms leading up to hospital admission, these were consistent with stable angina, but have not recurred after discharge home. She maintains a reasonably active lifestyle, and has not noted any adverse effects from her therapy. You decide to prescribe simvastatin 20 mg nightly in addition to her existing medications. Rather puzzled, the patient suggests that her cholesterol had previously been described as "ok" by the attending physician and after a health screen by her GP 1 year ago.

66 The patient suggests that her cholesterol had previously been described as 'ok' by the attending physician 99

Management issues

- Our understanding of the contribution of hypercholesterolaemia to overall cardiovascular risk has evolved rapidly over recent years. Once viewed simply as a marker of risk, it emerged as having an important causal role.
- It is impossible to define cut-off values for "abnormal" cholesterol concentrations because of their normal distribution in large populations. Therefore, attempts have been made to identify clinical action limits so that a target group requiring therapy might be defined on the basis of an absolute total or LDL-cholesterol value.
- Current data support the view that cholesterol reduction lowers risk, regardless of baseline concentrations, and no minimum optimum cholesterol concentration has been identified.
- With this in mind, cholesterol-lowering therapy should be introduced in patients at high cardiovascular risk. Often this will mean treating patients with "average" or "below average" baseline cholesterol concentrations. Treatment is therefore indicated on the basis of overall cardiovascular risk in most patients, rather than absolute cholesterol concentrations alone.
- In patients with established cardiovascular disease or diabetes mellitus, as illustrated in this case, therapy is indicated without resort to estimation of future cardiovascular risk.

66 Cholesterol reduction lowers risk, regardless of baseline concentrations 99

66 Cholesterol-lowering therapy should be introduced in patients at high cardiovascular risk 99

Follow-up

This patient had a 10-year cardiovascular risk of around 23%, based on her current smoking status, blood pressure of 152/88 mmHg before treatment, total cholesterol 5.5 mmol/L, and HDL-cholesterol 1.0 mmol/L. Six weeks after initiation of simvastatin 20 mg, total cholesterol had fallen to 3.8 mmol/L and the dose of treatment was escalated to

125

simvastatin 40 mg nightly. Blood pressure in clinic averaged 148/86 mmHg, despite atenolol, and, therefore, lisinopril 10 mg daily was introduced. Follow-up after a further 8 weeks showed total cholesterol 3.4 mmol/L, estimated LDL-cholesterol 2.3 mmol/L, blood pressure 142/80 mmHg and, unfortunately, the patient had continued to smoke despite encouragement to quit.

Case study 4

Poor drug compliance

A 64-year-old man is admitted to hospital for elective right knee joint replacement for severe osteoarthritis. He has a past history of diabetes mellitus and hypertension, and takes metformin 1 g twice daily, aspirin 75 mg daily, lisinopril 20 mg daily, amlodipine 10 mg daily, doxazosin 8 mg daily, furosemide 40 mg daily, and co-codamol (500 mg/8 mg) 8 tablets per day. You are asked to review him because shortly before he was due to be transferred to theatre for surgery he is noted to be profoundly hypotensive. Ambulatory pre-operative assessment 1 week earlier found blood pressure 156/82 mmHg. On reviewing his casenotes you note that his blood pressure on arrival in the ward on the previous evening was recorded at 168/86 mmHg. His normal medications had been administered at 8 am and 3 hours later his blood pressure was recorded as 104/56 mmHg. Resting pulse rate is 84 per minute, and an ECG is normal.

&&Shortly before he was due to be transferred to theatre for surgery he is noted to be profoundly hypotensive 99

&&Patients might require considerable encouragement to admit they are not taking their regular therapy as instructed 99

Management issues

- **Drug compliance may be a major difficulty for a large number of patients receiving multiple combination therapies to reduce cardiovascular risk.**
- **Compliance is often difficult to measure objectively, and patients might require considerable encouragement to admit that they are not taking their regular therapy as instructed.**
- **Education should enable patients to understand why multiple medications are often required, and to understand the long-term benefits of treatment.**
- **Compliance is less likely to be achieved in patients who require complicated regimens, involving multiple daily administrations, and where adverse effects occur.**
- **Adverse effects of antihypertensive drugs are more likely in the setting of erratic use or after initial introduction.**

- Patients should be encouraged to persist with therapy with regular dosing intervals if possible.
- Drug administration in hospital is by no means failsafe either, because this is rarely directly supervised.
- It may be easier to establish non-compliance by means of directly observed drug therapy in a controlled environment or, rarely, by direct demonstration of drug in blood or urine samples.
- An alternative possibility that needs consideration is that different formulations of drug had been administered. This is particularly relevant for sustained-release preparations that can vary substantially. However, in this patient, the formulation administered was identical to his home supply.

❝ Patients should be encouraged to persist with therapy ❞

Follow-up

This patient was discharged home with blood pressure 136/78 mmHg, and his antihypertensive drugs were reduced to lisinopril 20 mg daily, amlodipine 5 mg daily, furosemide 40 mg daily. Unfortunately, his operation had to be rescheduled to a later date.

Case study 5

Metabolic syndrome

A 46-year-old woman is referred to the local Hypertension Clinic. She has a history of obesity and hypertension treated for the past 5 years, and is currently receiving bendroflumethiazide 2.5 mg daily, long-acting nifedipine 30 mg daily and inhaled salbutamol when required for asthma. Her GP has found her blood pressure consistently elevated, but she has been intolerant of added doxazosin. She has never used tobacco. Her father died after an MI, aged 52 years. On examination, blood pressure is 132/94 mmHg, weight is 99 kg, BMI 37.3 kg/m², and there is mild ankle oedema. Urinalysis shows a trace of proteinuria only, and ECG is normal. Laboratory investigations show random glucose 8.2 mmol/L, total cholesterol 5.6 mmol/L, HDL-cholesterol 0.9 mmol/L, triglycerides 6.8 mmol/L, urea 4.8 mmol/L, creatinine 88 µmol/L, and urate 436 µmol/L.

❝ Her GP has found her blood pressure consistently elevated ❞

127

> *Patients with impaired glucose tolerance are at very high risk of developing type 2 diabetes*

Management issues

- This patient has hypertension in the context of obesity and possible metabolic syndrome, based on her very high BMI and abnormally high random glucose, triglyceride and urate concentrations. Liver biochemistry, fasting glucose and fasting lipid profile should be checked.
- Patients with impaired glucose tolerance are at very high risk of developing type 2 diabetes. Management involves patient education, with a strong emphasis on lifestyle measures and weight loss to delay progression to overt diabetes.
- There has been significant debate over the contribution of thiazide-type diuretics to insulin resistance. In the low doses required for blood pressure lowering, metabolic complications are uncommon but might make a small contribution in patients with an underlying predisposition to insulin resistance syndrome.
- In the short term, blood pressure control is likely to require escalation of therapy by addition of an ACE inhibitor or AIIRA. This should be adopted in the context of a concerted effort to lose weight, and the combined effects on blood pressure response should be closely monitored. The adverse developmental effects of these drugs on the foetus should be borne in mind when considering their use in women of child-bearing age.
- If patients are able to demonstrate sufficient motivation to lose weight by lifestyle modification, then consideration should be given to adjunctive pharmacological treatments to aid weight loss. In patients with features of metabolic syndrome, orlistat might be a preferred agent due to its ability to favourably modify serum glucose and triglyceride concentrations, blood pressure and insulin sensitivity.

> *Blood pressure control is likely to require escalation of therapy by addition of an ACE inhibitor or AIIRA*

> *In patients with features of metabolic syndrome, orlistat might be a preferred agent to aid weight loss*

Follow-up

This patient had fasting glucose 6.8 mmol/L, and was given encouragement to lose weight by way of dietary and lifestyle modification. She was prescribed losartan 50 mg daily to take in addition to the thiazide and calcium channel blocker. Eight weeks later, she reported no adverse effects, average clinic blood pressure was 126/88 mmHg, and weight had increased to 102 kg! Further encouragement was given to lose weight and a formal dietitian review was arranged. The dose of her long-acting nifedipine preparation was increased to 60 mg daily.

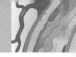

Abbreviations

Conditions

CAD	Coronary artery disease
CHD	Coronary heart disease
CHF	Congestive heart failure
CVD	Cardiovascular disease
ESRD	End-stage renal disease
HD	Heart disease
HHD	Hypertensive heart disease
IFG	Impaired fasting glucose
IGT	Impaired glucose tolerance
ISH	Isolated systolic hypertension
LBBB	Left bundle branch block
LVH	Left ventricular hypertrophy
MI	Myocardial infarction
PVD	Peripheral vascular disease

Drugs and molecules

ACE	Angiotensin converting enzyme
AIIRA	Angiotensin II receptor antagonist
CB1	Cannabinoid-1 receptor
COCP	Combined oral contraceptive pill
CRP	C-reactive protein
DPP IV	Dipeptidyl peptidase IV
GLP-1	Glucagon-like protein-1
HbA_{1c}	Glycosylated haemoglobin
HDL	High-density lipoprotein
HMG-CoA	3-hydroxy-3-methylglutaryl coenzyme A
HRT	Hormone replacement therapy
IPP	Isoleucine-proline-proline
LDL	Low-density lipoprotein
MAOI	Monoamine oxidase inhibitor
PAI-1	Plasminogen activator inhibitor-1
PPAR	Peroxisome proliferators-activated receptor
TSH	Thyroid-stimulating hormone
VLDL	Very low-density lipoprotein
VMA	Vanillylmandelic acid
VPP	Valine-proline-proline

Examinations and measurements

ABPM	Ambulatory blood pressure measurement
BMI	Body mass index

BP	Blood pressure
DBP	Diastolic blood pressure
ECG	Electrocardiogram
FPG	Fasting plasma glucose
hsCRP	High-sensitivity C-reactive protein
SBP	Systolic blood pressure
TC	Total cholesterol

Organizations and guidelines

AAMI	Association for the Advancement of Medical Instrumentation
ACC	American College of Cardiology
ACCP	American College of Chest Physicians
AHA	American Heart Association
BHS	British Hypertension Society
CCS	Canadian Cardiovascular Society
EGSIR	European Group for the Study of Insulin Resistance
ESC	European Society of Cardiology
FDA	Food and Drug Administration
IDF	International Diabetes Federation
JBS-2	Joint British Societies guidelines for cardiovascular risk reduction
JNC VII	Joint National Committee on Prevention, Detection, Evaluation, and Treatment of High Blood Pressure guidelines (version 7)
NCEP	National Cholesterol Education Program
NHBLI	National Heart, Lung, and Blood Institute
NHS	National Health Service
SCORE	Systemic COronary Risk Evaluation
WHO	World Health Organization

Other

A&E	Accident and Emergency department
CABG	Coronary artery bypass graft
CI	Confidence interval
HR	Hazard ratio
LOCF	Last observation carried forward
OR	Odds ratio
RR	Risk reduction
RRR	Relative risk reduction

Trials

4S	Scandinavian Simvastatin Survival Study
AFCAPS/TexCAPS	Air Force/Texas Coronary Atherosclerosis Prevention Study
ALLHAT	Antihypertensive and Lipid-Lowering Treatment to Prevent Heart Attack Trial
ANBP-2	Second Australian National Blood Pressure
ASCOT-LLA	Anglo-Scandinavian Cardiac Outcomes Trial – Lipid Lowering Arm
CAPRIE	Clopidogrel vs Aspirin in patients at Risk of Ischemic Events
CHARISMA	Clopidogrel for High Atherothrombotic Risk and Ischemic Stabilization, Management, and Avoidance
CURE	Clopidogrel in Unstable Angina to prevent Recurrent Events
DAIS	Diabetes Atherosclerosis Intervention Study
DREAM	Diabetes Risk Assessment and Microalbuminuria study
EUROPA	European Trial on Reduction of Cardiac Events with Perindopril in Stable Coronary Artery Disease
FACET	Fosinopril Versus Amlodipine Cardiovascular Events Randomised Trial
GATE	Glitazones and the Endothelium
GEMINI	Glycemic Effects in Diabetes Mellitus Carvedilol-Metopolol Comparison in Hypertensives
GRACE	Global Registry of Acute Coronary Events
HERS	Heart and Estrogen/progestin Replacement Study
HOPE	Heart Outcomes Prevention Evaluation Study
HOT	Hypertension Optimal Treatment
HPS	Heart Protection Study
IDNT	Irbesartan Diabetic Nephropathy Trial
INSIGHT	International Nifedipine-GITS Study: Intervention as a Goal in Hypertension Treatment
INTERHEART	Global Study of Risk Factors in Acute Myocardial Infarction
IRMA II	Irbesartan Microalbuminuria II
LIFE	Losartan Intervention For Endpoint reduction in hypertension

MONICA	Monitoring trends and determinants in cardio-vascular disease
MRFIT	Multiple Risk Factors Intervention Trial
ONTARGET	Ongoing Telmisartan Alone and in Combination with Ramipril Global Endpoint Trial
PIONEER	PPARγ Activation Results in Overall Improvement of Clinical and Metabolic Markers Associated with Insulin Resistance Independent of Long-term Glucose Control
PROactive	Prospective Pioglitazone Clinical Trial in Macrovascular Events Study
PRoFESS	Prevention Regimen for Effectively Avoiding Second Strokes
PROSPER	PROspective study of Pravastatin in Elderly individuals at Risk of vascular disease
RECORD	Rosiglitazone Evaluated for Cardiac Outcomes and Regulation of Glycaemia in Diabetes
RENAAL	Reduction of Endpoints in Non-Insulin Dependent Diabetes Mellitus with the Angiotensin II Antagonist Losartan
RIO	Rimonabant in Obesity
SHEP	Systolic Hypertension in the Elderly Program
STOP-2	Swedish Trial in Old Patients with Hypertension 2 Ongoing trial
STOP-Hypertension	Swedish Trial in Old Patients with Hypertension
Syst-Eur	Systolic Hypertension in Europe
UKPDS	UK Prospective Diabetes Study
VA-HIT	Veterans Affairs High-Density Lipoprotein Cholesterol Intervention Trial
VALUE	Valsartan Antihypertensive Long-term Use Evaluation
WHI	Women's Health Initiative
WOSCOPS	West of Scotland Coronary Prevention Study

Contact information for useful organizations

Action on Smoking and Health
2013 H Street, N. W., Wash., DC 20006, USA
Tel: +1 202 659 4310
Website: http://www.ash.org

American College of Cardiology
Heart House, 9111 Old Georgetown Road, Bethesda,
MD 20814-1699, USA
Tel: +1 800 253 4636, ext. 694   Fax: +1 301 897 9745
Website: http://www.acc.org

American College of Chest Physicians
3300 Dundee Road, Northbrook, Illinois 60062-2348, USA
Tel: +1 847 498 1400
Website: http://www.chestnet.org

American Diabetes Association
(Attn: National Call Center), 1701 North Beauregard Street,
Alexandria, VA 22311, USA
Tel: +1 800 342 2383
Website: http://www.diabetes.org

American Heart Association
One North Franklin, Chicago, IL 60606-3421, USA
Tel: +1 312 422 3000
Website: http://www.aha.org

American Society of Hypertension
148 Madison Avenue, New York, NY 10016, USA
Tel: +1 212 696 9099   Fax: +1 212 696 0711
E-mail: ash@ash-us.org
Website: http://www.ash-us.org

Association for Research into Arterial Structure and Physiology (ARTERY)
ARTERY Secretariat, 113-119 High Street, Middlesex, TW12 1NJ, UK
Tel: +44 (0)20 8979 8300   Fax: +44 (0)20 8979 6700
E-mail: artery@hamptonmedical.com
Website: www.artery.ukevents.org

British Cardiovascular Society
9 Fitzroy Square, London W1T 5HW, UK
Tel: +44 (0)20 7383 3887   Fax: +44 (0)20 7388 0903
E-mail: enquiries@bcs.com
Website: http://www.bcs.com

133

British Heart Foundation
14 Fitzhardinge Street, London W1H 6DH, UK
Tel: +44 (0)20 7935 0185   Fax: +44 (0)20 7486 5820
E-mail: internet@bhf.org.uk
Website: http://www.bhf.org.uk

British Hypertension Society
BHS Administrative Officer, Leicester Royal Infirmary, LE2 7LX, UK
Tel: +44 (0)7717 467 973
E-mail: bhs@le.ac.uk
Website: http://www.bhsoc.org

Consensus Action on Salt and Health (CASH)
Blood Pressure Unit, Department of Medicine, St George's, University of London, Cranmer Terrace, London SW17 0RE, UK
E-mail: cash@sgul.ac.uk
Website: http://www.actiononsalt.org.uk

Diabetes UK
10 Parkway, London NW1 7AA, UK
Tel: +44 (0)20 7424 1000   Fax: +44 (0)20 7424 1001
E-mail: info@diabetes.org.uk
Website: http://www.diabetes.org.uk

European Atherosclerosis Society
Executive Office, Altonagatan 7, SE 211 38 Malmö, Sweden
Tel: +46 40 240 750   Fax: +46 40 240 751
E-mail: info@eas-society.org
Website: http://www.eas-society.org

European Council for Cardiovascular Research
ECCR Secretariat, 113-119 High Street, Middlesex, TW12 1NJ, UK
Tel: +44 (0)20 8979 8300   Fax: +44 (0)20 8979 6700
E-mail: eccr@hamptonmedical.com
Website: http://www.eccr.org

European Society of Cardiology
The European Heart House, 2035 Route des Colles, B.P. 179 – Les Templiers, FR-06903 Sophia Antipolis, France
Tel: +33 4 92 94 76 00   Fax: +33 4 92 94 76 01
Website: http://www.escardio.org

European Society of Hypertension
E-mail: info@eshonline.org
Website: http://www.eshonline.org

Global Prevention Alliance
Website: http://www.preventionalliance.net/index.htm

Heart UK
7 North Road, Maidenhead, Berkshire SL6 1PE, UK
Tel: +44 (0)1628 628 638   Fax: +44 (0)1628 628 698
E-mail: ask@heartuk.org.uk
Website: http://www.heartuk.org.uk

High Blood Pressure Research Council of Australia
HBPRCA Secretariat, 4/184 Main Street, Lilydale, VIC 3140, Australia
Tel: +61 3 9739 7697   Fax +61 3 9739 7076
E-mail: hbprca@meetingsfirst.com.au
Website: http://www.hbprca.com.au

International Atherosclerosis Society
E-mail: info@athero.org
Website: http://www.athero.org

International Diabetes Federation (IDF)
Avenue Emile De Mot 19, B-1000 Brussels, Belgium
Tel: +32 2 5385511   Fax: +32 2 5385114
E-mail: info@idf.org
Website: http://www.idf.org

International Obesity Taskforce
231 North Gower Street, London NW1 2NR, UK
Tel: +44 (0)20 7691 1900   Fax: +44 (0)20 7387 6033
E-mail: obesity@iotf.org
Website: http://www.iotf.org

International Society of Hypertension
ISH Secretariat, 113-119 High Street, Middlesex, TW12 1NJ, UK
Tel: +44 (0)20 8979 8300   Fax: +44 (0)20 8979 6700
E-mail: secretariat@ish-world.com
Website: http://www.ish-world.com

Primary Care Cardiovascular Society
36 Berrymede Road, London W4 5JD, UK
Tel: +44 (0)20 8994 8775   Fax: +44 (0)20 8742 2130
E-mail: office@pccs.org.uk
Website: http://www.pccs.org.uk

World Heart Federation
5, avenue du Mail, 1205 Geneva, Switzerland
Tel: +41 22 807 03 20   Fax: +41 22 807 03 39
E-mail: admin@worldheart.org
Website: http://www.worldheart.org

World Hypertension League
Website: http://www.meduohio.edu/whl/index.html

References

1. Murray CJL, Lopez AD. Mortality by cause for eight regions of the world. Global burden of disease study. Lancet 1997;349:1269–1276.
2. Murray CJL, Lopez AD. Alternative projections of mortality and global burden of disease study. Lancet 1997;349:1498–1504.
3. World Health Organization. The World Health Report 2004 – Changing History. Geneva: WHO, 2004.
4. Petersen S, Peto V, Rayner M, et al. European Cardiovascular Disease Statistics. London: British Heart Foundation, 2005. http://www.heartstats.org/temp/Tabsp13.2spweb05.xls [accessed February 2006].
5. Lloyd-Jones DM, Larson MG, Beiser A, Levy D. Lifetime risk of developing coronary heart disease. Lancet 1999;353:89–92.
6. Office for National Statistics. The Health of Adult Britain. London: The Stationery Office, 1997.
7. Petersen S, Peto V, Scarborough P, Rayner M. Coronary Heart Disease Statistics. London: British Heart Foundation, 2005.
8. Unal B, Critchley JA, Capewell S. Explaining the decline in coronary heart disease mortality in England and Wales between 1981 and 2000. Circulation 2004;109:1101–1107.
9. National Heart, Lung, and Blood Institute. Morbidity and Mortality: 1996 Chartbook on Cardiovascular, Lung, and Blood Diseases. Bethesda, MD: National Institutes of Health, 1996.
10. Hunink MG, Goldman L, Tosteson AN, et al. The recent decline in mortality from coronary heart disease, 1980–90. The effect of secular trends in risk factors and treatment. JAMA 1997;277:535–542.
11. World Health Organization Mortality Statistics at http://www3.who.int/whosis/menu.cfm?path=whosis,mort&language=english [accessed February 2006].
12. Tunstall-Pedoe H, Kuulasmaa K, Mahonen M, et al. Contribution of trends in survival and coronary-event rates in changes in coronary heart disease mortality: 10-year results from 37 WHO MONICA project populations. Lancet 1999;353:1547–1557.
13. Publications from the WHO Monica project. http://www.ktl.fi/publications/monica/index.html [accessed February 2006].
14. Kuulasmaa K, Tunstall-Pedoe H, Dobson A, et al. Estimation of contribution of changes in classic risk factors to trends in coronary-event rates across the WHO MONICA project populations. Lancet 2000;355:675–887.
15. Lacey L, Tabberer M. Economic burden of post-acute myocardial infarction heart failure in the United Kingdom. Eur J Heart Fail 2005;7:677–683.
16. American Heart Association. Heart Disease and Stroke Statistics: 2004 Update. Dallas, Texas: American Heart Association, 2004.
17. Stampfer MJ, Hu FB, Manson JE, et al. Primary prevention of coronary heart disease in women through diet and lifestyle. N Engl J Med 2000;343:16–22.
18. Yusuf S, Hawken S, Ounpuu S, et al; INTERHEART Study Investigators. Effect of potentially modifiable risk factors associated with myocardial infarction in 52 countries (the INTERHEART study): case-control study. Lancet 2004;364:937–952.
19. Hennekens CH. Increasing burden of cardiovascular disease: current knowledge and future directions for research on risk factors. Circulation 1998;97:1095–1102.
20. Wolf PA. Prevention of stroke. Lancet 1998;352(suppl 3):SIII15–SIII18.
21. Kannel W. The Framingham study. BMJ 1976;2:1255.
22. Anderson K, Wilson P, Odell P, Kannel W. An updated coronary risk profile. A statement for health professionals. Circulation 1991;83:356–362.
23. Stamler J, Wentworth D, Neaton J. Is relationship between serum cholesterol and risk of premature death from coronary heart disease continuous and graded? Findings in 356,222 primary screenees of the Multiple Risk Factor Intervention Trial (MRFIT). JAMA 1986;256:2823–2828.
24. Grundy S. Statin trials and goals of cholesterol-lowering therapy. Circulation 1998;97:1436–1439.
25. Stamler J, Stamler R, Neaton J. Blood pressure, systolic and diastolic, and cardiovascular risks. US population data. Arch Intern Med 1993;153:598–615.
26. Haffner S, Lehto S, Ronnemaa T, et al. Mortality from coronary heart disease in subjects with type 2 diabetes and in nondiabetic subjects with and without prior myocardial infarction. N Engl J Med 1998;339:229–234.
27. Rantala A, Kauma H, Lilja M, et al. Prevalence of the metabolic syndrome in drug-treated hypertensive patients and control subjects. J Intern Med 1999;245:163–174.
28. Fodor JG, Frohlich JJ, Genest JJG, McPherson PR, for the Working Group on Hypercholesterolemia and Other Dyslipidemias. Recommendations for the management and treatment of dyslipidemia. CMAJ 2000;162(10):1441–1447.
29. Perreault S, Dorais M, Coupal L, et al. Impact of treating hyperlipidemia or hypertension to reduce the risk of death from coronary artery disease. CMAJ 1999;160:1449–1455.
30. Pollini G, Maugeri U, Tringali S, et al. Prevalence of hypertension and cardiovascular risk factors in workers of petrochemical industry. The Pavia Study. G Ital Med Lav 1986;8:89–108.
31. Stern N, Grosskopf I, Shapira I, et al. Risk factor clustering in hypertensive patients: impact of the reports of NCEP-II and second joint task force on coronary prevention on JNC-VI guidelines. J Intern Med 2000;248:203–210.
32. Williams RR, Hunt SC, Hopkins PN, et al. Familial dyslipidemic hypertension. Evidence from 58 Utah families for a syndrome present in approximately 12% of patients with essential hypertension. JAMA 1988;259:3579–3586.

33. Reaven GM. Role of insulin resistance in human disease. Diabetes 1988;37:1595–1600.
34. Meigs J. Epidemiology of the metabolic syndrome, 2002. Am J Manag Care 2002;8:S283–S292.
35. Reaven G. Metabolic syndrome: pathophysiology and implications for management of cardiovascular disease. Circulation 2002;106:268–286.
36. Reaven GM. Pathophysiology of insulin resistance in human disease. Physiol Rev 1995;75:473–486.
37. Alberti KG, Zimmet P. Definition, diagnosis and classification of diabetes mellitus and its complications. Part 1: diagnosis and classification of diabetes mellitus provisional report of a WHO consultation. Diabet Med 1998;15:539–553.
38. Balkau B, Charles MA. Comment on the provisional report from the WHO consultation. European Group for the Study of Insulin Resistance (EGIR). Diabet Med 1999;16:442–443.
39. Laaksonen DE, Lakka HM, Niskanen LK, et al. Metabolic syndrome and development of diabetes mellitus: application and validation of recently suggested definitions of the metabolic syndrome in a prospective cohort study. Am J Epidemiol 2002;156:1070–1077.
40. Lakka HM, Laaksonen DE, Lakka TA, et al. The metabolic syndrome and total and cardiovascular disease mortality in middle-aged men. JAMA 2002;288:2709–2716.
41. International Diabetes Federation. The IDF consensus worldwide definition of the metabolic syndrome. Brussels: IDF, 2005.
42. Executive Summary of the Third Report of the National Cholesterol Education Program (NCEP) Expert Panel on Detection, Evaluation, and Treatment of High Blood Cholesterol in Adults. JAMA 2001;285:2486–2497.
43. Haffner SM. Epidemiology of insulin resistance and its relation to coronary artery disease. Am J Cardiol 1999;84:11J–14J.
44. Juhan-Vague I, Alessi MC, Morange PE. Hypofibrinolysis and increased PAI-1 are linked to atherothrombosis via insulin resistance and obesity. Ann Med 2000;32:78–84.
45. Koenig W. Insulin resistance, heart disease and inflammation. Identifying the 'at-risk' patient: the earlier the better? The role of inflammatory markers. Int J Clin Pract Suppl 2002;132:23–30.
46. Ukkola O, Santaniemi M. Adiponectin: a link between excess adiposity and associated comorbidities? J Mol Med 2002;80:696–702.
47. Montagnani M, Quon MJ. Insulin action in vascular endothelium: potential mechanisms linking insulin resistance with hypertension. Diabetes Obes Metab 2000;2:285–292.
48. Avramoglu RK, Qiu W, Adeli K. Mechanisms of metabolic dyslipidemia in insulin resistant states: deregulation of hepatic and intestinal lipoprotein secretion. Front Biosci 2003;8:D464–D476.
49. de Jongh S, Lilien MR, op't Roodt J, et al. Early statin therapy restores endothelial function in children with familial hypercholesterolemia. J Am Coll Cardiol 2002;40:2117–2121.
50. Scandinavian Simvastatin Survival Study Group. Randomised trial of cholesterol lowering in 4444 patients with coronary heart disease: the Scandinavian Simvastatin Survival Study (4S). Lancet 1994;344:1383–1389.
51. The Cholesterol and Recurrent Events Trial Investigators. The effect of pravastatin on coronary events after myocardial infarction in patients with average cholesterol levels. N Engl J Med 1996;335:1001–1009.
52. The Long-Term Intervention with Pravastatin Group in Ischaemic Disease (LIPID) Study Group. Prevention of cardiovascular events and death with pravastatin in patients with coronary heart disease and a broad range of initial cholesterol levels. N Engl J Med 1998;339:1349–1357.
53. Athyros VG, Papageorgiou AA, Mercouris BR. The GREek Atorvastatin and Coronary heart disease Evaluation (GREACE) Study. Curr Med Res Opin 2002;18:220–228.
54. Heart Protection Study Collaborative Group. MRC/BHF Heart Protection Study of cholesterol lowering with simvastatin in 20 536 high-risk individuals: a randomised placebo-controlled trial. Lancet 2002;360:7–22.
55. Anderson KM, Odell PM, Wilson PWF, Kannel WB. Cardiovascular disease risk profiles. Am Heart J 1991;121:293–298.
56. Haq IU, Jackson PR. Sheffield risk and treatment table for cholesterol lowering for primary prevention of coronary heart disease. Lancet 1995;346:1467–1471.
57. Jackson R. Updated New Zealand cardiovascular disease risk-benefit prediction guide. BMJ 2000;320:709–710.
58. Payne R. The University of Edinburgh Cardiovascular Risk Calculator. http://cvrisk.mvm.ed.ac.uk/calculator.htm [accessed February 2006].
59. Global Registry of Acute Coronary Events (GRACE). Center for Outcomes Research, University of Massachusetts Medical School. http://www.outcomes-umassmed.org/grace/acs_risk.cfm [accessed February 2006].
60. Eagle KA, Lim MJ, Dabbous OH, et al; for the GRACE Investigators. A validated prediction model for all forms of acute coronary syndrome: estimating the risk of 6-month postdischarge death in an international registry. JAMA 2004;291:2727–2733.
61. Conroy RM, Pyörälä AP, Fitzgerald AP. Estimation of ten-year risk of fatal cardiovascular disease in Europe: the SCORE project. Eur Heart J 2003;24:987–1003.
62. Joint British Societies. JBS-2: Joint British Societies' guidelines on prevention of cardiovascular disease in clinical practice. Heart 2005;91(suppl 5):v1–52.
63. Valler-Jones T, Wedgbury K. Measuring blood pressure using the mercury sphygmomanometer. Br J Nurs 2005;14:145–150.
64. O'Leary DH, Polak JF, Kronmal RA, et al. Carotid-artery intima and media thickness as a risk factor for myocardial infarction and stroke in older adults. Cardiovascular Health Study Collaborative Research Group. N Engl J Med 1999;340:14–22.

137

65. Criqui MH, Langer RD, Fronek A, et al. Mortality over a period of 10 years in patients with peripheral arterial disease. N Engl J Med 1992;326:381–386.

66. Kuller LH, Shemanski L, Psaty BM, et al. Sub-clinical disease as an independent risk factor for cardiovascular disease. Circulation 1995;92:720–726.

67. Leng GC, Fowkes FGR, Lee AJ, et al. Use of ankle brachial pressure index to predict cardiovascular events and death: a cohort study. BMJ 1996;313:1440–1444.

68. Wenger NK. Coronary heart disease: an older woman's major health risk. BMJ 1997;315:1085–1090.

69. Knopp RH. Risk factors for coronary artery disease in women. Am J Cardiol 2002;89(suppl):28E–35E.

70. Hu FB, Grodstein F. Post-menopausal hormone therapy and the risk of cardiovascular disease: the epidemiologic evidence. Am J Cardiol 2002;90(suppl):26F–29F.

71. Collins P. Clinical cardiovascular studies of hormone replacement therapy. Am J Cardiol 2002;90(suppl):30F–34F.

72. Grady D, Rubin SM, Petitti DB, et al. Hormone therapy to prevent disease and prolong life in post-menopausal women. Ann Intern Med 1992;117:1016–1037.

73. Stamfer MJ, Colditz GA. Estrogen replacement therapy and coronary heart disease: a quantitative assessment of the epidemiologic evidence. Prev Med 1991;20:47–55.

74. Writing Group for WHI Investigators. Risks and benefits of estrogen plus progestin in healthy postmenopausal women. Principal results from the Women's Health Initiative randomized controlled trial. JAMA 2002;288:321–333.

75. Hulley S, Grady D, Bush T, et al. Randomized trial of estrogen plus progestin for secondary prevention of coronary heart disease in postmenopausal women. JAMA 1998;280:605–613.

76. Berenson GS, McMahan CA, Voors AW, et al. Cardiovascular Risk Factors in Children: The Early Natural History of Atherosclerosis and Essential Hypertension. New York: Oxford University Press, 1980.

77. Berenson GS, editor. Causation of Cardiovascular Risk Factors in Children: Perspectives on Cardiovascular Risk in Early Life. New York: Raven Press, 1986.

78. Berenson GS, Srinivasan S, Nicklas T. Atherosclerosis: a nutritional disease of childhood. Am J Cardiol 1998;82:22T–29T.

79. Wissler RW, Strong JP, PDAY Research Group. Risk factors and progression of atherosclerosis in youth. Am J Pathol 1998;153:1023–1033.

80. Mahoney LH, Burns TL, Stanford W, et al. Coronary risk factors measured in childhood and young adult life are associated with coronary artery calcification in young adults. J Am Coll Cardiol 1996;27:277–284.

81. Joseph A, Ackerman D, Talley JD, et al. Manifestations of coronary atherosclerosis in young trauma victims – an autopsy study. J Am Coll Cardiol 1993;22:459–467.

82. Burt VL, Whelton P, Roccella EJ, et al. Prevalence of hypertension in US adult population: results from Third National Health and Nutrition Examination Study. Hypertension 1995;25:303–313.

83. Staessen JA, Fagard R, Thijs L, et al. Randomised double-blind comparison of placebo and active treatment for older patients with isolated systolic hypertension: the Systolic Hypertension in Europe (Syst-Eur) Trial Investigators. Lancet 1997;350:757–764.

84. Staessen JA, Gasowski J, Wang JG, et al. Risks of untreated and treated isolated systolic hypertension in the elderly: meta-analysis of outcome trials. Lancet 2000;355:865–873.

85. Downs JR, Clearfield SM, Weis S, et al; for AFCAPS/TexasCAPS Research Group. Primary prevention of acute coronary events with lovastatin in men and women with average cholesterol levels. JAMA 1998;279:1615–1622.

86. Shepherd J, Blauw GJ, Murphy MB, et al. Pravastatin in elderly individuals at risk of vascular disease (PROSPER): a randomised controlled trial. Lancet 2002;360:1623–1630.

87. Pan XR, Li GW, Hu YH, et al. Effects of diet and exercise in preventing NIDDM in people with impaired glucose tolerance. The Da Qing IGT and Diabetes Study. Diabetes Care 1997;20:537–544.

88. Tuomilehto J. Controlling glucose and blood pressure in type 2 diabetes. BMJ 2001;7250:394–395.

89. Pownall HJ. Alcohol: lipid metabolism and cardioprotection. Curr Atheroscler Rep 2002;4:107–112.

90. Kaplan NM. The deadly quartet. Arch Intern Med 1989;149:1514–1520.

91. Miller PM, Anton RF, Egan BM, et al. Excessive alcohol consumption and hypertension: clinical implications of current research. J Clin Hypertens 2005;7:346–351.

92. Burr ML, Fehily AM, Gilbert JF, et al. Effects of changes in fat, fish, and fibre intakes on death and myocardial reinfarction: diet and reinfarction trial (DART). Lancet 1989;2:757–761.

93. Gruppo Italiano per lo Studio della Sopravvivenza nell'Infarto miocardico. Dietary supplementation with n-3 polyunsaturated fatty acids and vitamin E after myocardial infarctionL results of the GISSI-Prevenzione trial. Lancet 1999;354:447–55.

94. Marckmann P, Gronbaek M. Fish consumption and coronary heart disease mortality. A systemic review of prospective cohort studies. Eur J Clin Nutr 1999;53:585–590.

95. Campbell NRC. Will lifestyle modifications reduce blood pressure? Canadian Family Physician 1999;45:1640–1642.

96. Campbell NRC, Taylor G. Healthier lifestyles: bringing down blood pressure. Perspectives in Cardiology 1999;May:47–53.

97. Prochaska JO, DiClemente CC, Norcross JC. In search of how people change: applications to addictive behaviours. Diabetes Spectrum 1993;6:25–33.

98. Imperial Cancer Research Fund OXCHECK Study Group. Effectiveness of health checks conducted by nurses in primary care: results of the OXCHECK study after one year. BMJ 1994;308:308–312.

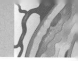

99. Family Heart Study Group. Randomised controlled trial evaluating cardiovascular screening and intervention in general practice: principal results of British family heart study. BMJ 1994;308:313–320.

100. Smith CJ, Livingston SD, Doolittle DJ. An international literature survey of IARC Group I carcinogens reported in mainstream cigarette smoke. Food Chem Toxicol 1997;35:1107–1130.

101. Hecht SS. Tobacco smoke carcinogens and lung cancer. J Natl Cancer Inst 1999;91:1194–1210.

102. Waring WS. The role of pharmacotherapy in assisting smoking cessation. Eur J Clin Pharmacol 2003;59:351–356.

103. Benowitz NL, Fitzgerald GA, Wilson M, et al. Nicotine effects on eicosanoid formation and hemostatic function–comparison of transdermal nicotine and cigarette-smoking. J Am Coll Cardiol 1993;22:1159–1167.

104. Piantadosi CA. Perspective: carbon monoxide poisoning. N Engl J Med 2002;347:1054–1055.

105. Benowitz NL, Gourlay SG. Cardiovascular toxicity of nicotine: implications for nicotine replacement therapy. J Am Coll Cardiol 1997;29:1422–1431.

106. Kannel WB, Dagostino RB, Belanger AJ. Fibrinogen, cigarette-smoking, and risk of cardiovascular disease: insights from the Framingham study. Am Heart J 1987;113:1006–1010.

107. Chiang VL, Castleden WM, Leahy MF. Detection of reversible platelet aggregates in the blood of smokers and ex-smokers with peripheral vascular disease. Med J Aust 1992;156:601–603.

108. Pilz H, Oguogho A, Chehne F, et al. Quitting cigarette smoking results in a fast improvement of in vivo oxidation injury determined via plasma, serum and urinary isoprostane. Thromb Res 2000;99:209–221.

109. Rosenberg L, Kaufman DW, Helmrich SP, Shapiro S. The risk of myocardial infarction after quitting smoking in men under 55 years of age. N Engl J Med 1985;313:1511–1514.

110. Perkins J, Dick TB. Smoking and myocardial infarction: secondary prevention. Postgrad Med J 1985;61:295–300.

111. Kawachi I, Colditz GA, Stampfer MJ, et al. Smoking cessation in relation to total mortality rates in women. A prospective cohort study. Ann Intern Med 1993;119:992–1000.

112. Hughes JR, Gulliver SB, Fenwick JW, et al. Smoking cessation among self-quitters. Health Psychol 1992;11:331–334.

113. Stanton WR. DSM-III-R tobacco dependence and quitting during late adolescence. Addict Behav 1995;20:595–603.

114. Ascher JA, Cole JO, Colin JN, et al. Bupropion: a review of its mechanism of antidepressant activity. J Clin Psychiatry 1995;56:395–401.

115. Hurt RD, Sachs DP, Glover ED, et al. A comparison of sustained-release bupropion and placebo for smoking cessation. N Engl J Med 1997;337:1195–1202.

116. Jorenby DE, Leischow SJ, Nides MA, et al. A controlled trial of sustained-release bupropion, a nicotine patch, or both for smoking cessation. N Engl J Med 1999;340:685–691.

117. Doggrell SA. Clinical evidence for drug treatments in obesity-associated hypertensive patients—a discussion paper. Methods Find Exp Clin Pharmacol 2005;27:119–125.

118. Van Gaal LF, Rissanen AM, Scheen AJ, et al. Effects of the cannabinoid-1 receptor blocker rimonabant on weight reduction and cardiovascular risk factors in overweight patients: 1-year experience from the RIO-Europe study. Lancet 2005;365:1389–1397.

119. Pi-Sunyer FX, Aronne LJ, Heshmati HM, et al. Effect of rimonabant, a cannabinoid-1 receptor blocker, on weight and cardiometabolic risk factors in overweight or obese patients: RIO-North American: a randomized controlled trial. JAMA 2006;295:761–775.

120. Henningfield JE, Fant RV, Buchhalter AR, Stitzer ML. Pharmacotherapy for nicotine dependence. CA Cancer J Clin 2005;55:281–299.

121. Chakravarthy MV, Booth FW. Eating, exercise, and "thrifty" genotypes: connecting the dots toward an evolutionary understanding of modern chronic diseases. J Appl Physiol 2004;96:3–10.

122. American Diabetes Association Expert Panel. Type 2 diabetes in children and adolescents. Diabetes Care 2000;23:381–389.

123. Harris MI, Hadden WC, Knowler WC, Bennett PH. International criteria for the diagnosis of diabetes and impaired glucose tolerance. Diabetes Care 1985;8:562–567.

124. Adler AI, Neil HA, Manley SE, et al. Hyperglycemia and hyperinsulinemia at diagnosis of diabetes and their association with subsequent cardiovascular disease in the United Kingdom prospective diabetes study (UKPDS 47). Am Heart J 1999;138:S353–S359.

125. World Health Organization. Prevalence of diabetes in the WHO European region. http://www.who.int/diabetes/facts/world_figures/en/index4.html [accessed February 2006].

126. Wild S, Roglic G, Green A, et al. Global prevalence of diabetes: estimates for the year 2000 and projections for 2030. Diabetes Care 2004;27:1047–1053.

127. Roglic G, Unwin N, Bennett PH, et al. The burden of mortality attributable to diabetes: realistic estimates for the year 2000. Diabetes Care 2005;28:2130–2135.

128. Materson BJ, Preston RA. Prevention of diabetic nephropathy. Hosp Pract 1997;32:129–134.

129. United States Renal Data System (USRDS). Incidence and prevalence of ESRD. USRDS. Am J Kidney Dis 1997;30(2 suppl 1):S40–S53.

130. Haffner SM. Metabolic predictors of hypertension. J Hypertens 1999;17(suppl 3):S23–S28.

131. Gordois A, Scuffham P, Shearer A, Oglesby A. The health care costs of diabetic nephropathy in the United States and the United Kingdom. J Diab Complicat 2004;18:18–26.

132. Evans J, MacDonald T, Leese G, et al. Impact of type 1 and type 2 diabetes on patterns and costs of drug prescribing. Diabetes Care 2000;23:770–774.

133. Eastman R, Javitt J, Herman W, et al. Model of complications of NIDDM II: Analysis of the health benefits and cost-effectiveness of treating NIDDM with the goal of normoglycemia. Diabetes Care 1997;20:735–744.

134. Bakhai A, Collinson J, Flather MD, et al; for the PRAIS-UK Investigators. Diabetic patients with acute coronary syndromes in the UK: high risk and under treated. Results from the prospective registry of acute ischaemic syndromes in the UK (PRAIS-UK). Int J Cardiol 2005;100:79–84.

135. Orchard TJ, Forrest KY, Kuller LH, Becker DJ. Lipid and blood pressure treatment goals for type 1 diabetes: 10-year incidence data from the Pittsburgh Epidemiology of Diabetes Complications Study. Diabetes Care 2001;24:1053–1059.

136. Almdal T, Scharling H, Jensen JS, Vestergaard H. The independent effect of type 2 diabetes mellitus on ischemic heart disease, stroke, and death: a population-based study of 13,000 men and women with 20 years of follow-up. Arch Intern Med 2004;164:1422–1426.

137. Evans JMM, Wang J, Morris AD. Comparison of cardiovascular risk between patients with type 2 diabetes and those who had had a myocardial infarction: cross sectional and cohort studies. BMJ 2002;324:939–943.

138. Stratton IM, Adler AI, Neil HAW, et al. Association of glycemia with macrovascular and microvascular complications of type 2 diabetes (UKPDS 35): prospective observational studies. BMJ 2000;321:405–412.

139. Parving HH. Diabetic hypertensive patients. Is this a group in need of particular care and attention? Diabetes Care 1999;22(suppl 2):B76–B79.

140. Pahor M, Psaty BM, Alderman MH, et al. Therapeutic benefits of ACE inhibitors and other antihypertensive drugs in patients with type 2 diabetes. Diabetes Care 2000;23:888–892.

141. ALLHAT Collaborative Research Group. Major cardiovascular events in hypertensive patients randomized to doxazosin vs chlortalidone: the antihypertensive and lipid-lowering treatment to prevent heart attack trial (ALLHAT). JAMA 2000;283:1967–1975.

142. Report of the Expert Committee on the Diagnosis and Classification of Diabetes Mellitus. Diabetes Care 1997;20:1183–1197.

143. Behan KJ. Screening for diabetes: sensitivity and positive predictive value of risk factor total. Clin Lab Sci 2005;18:221–225.

144. The Diabetes Control and Complications (DCCT) Research Group. Effect of intensive therapy on the development and progression of diabetic nephropathy in the Diabetes Control and Complications Trial. Kidney Int 1995;47:1703–1720.

145. Young TK, Reading J, Elias B, O'Neil JD. Type 2 diabetes mellitus in Canada's first nations: status of an epidemic in progress. CMAJ 2000;163:561–566.

146. Howard BV, Lee ET, Cowan LD, et al. Rising tide of cardiovascular disease in American Indians. The Strong Heart Study. Circulation 1999;99:2389–2395.

147. Sairam K, Kulinskaya E, Bousgead GB, et al. Prevalence of undiagnosed diabetes mellitus in male erectile dysfunction. Br J Urol 2001;88:68–71.

148. Gerstein HC, Yusuf S, Holman R, et al; for the DREAM Trial Investigators. Rationale, design and recruitment characteristics of a large, simple international trial of diabetes prevention: the DREAM trial. Diabetologia 2004;47:1519–1527.

149. National Institute for Clinical Evidence. Clinical guidelines for type 2 diabetes: management of blood glucose. NICE 2002.

150. Franciosi M, Pellegrini F, De Berardis G, et al. The impact of blood glucose self-monitoring on metabolic control and quality of life in type 2 diabetic patients: an urgent need for better educational strategies. Diabetes Care 2001;24:1870–1877.

151. Gerstein HC. Dysglycaemia: a cardiovascular risk factor. Diabetes Res Clin Prac 1998;40(suppl):S9–S14.

152. UK Prospective Diabetes Study (UKPDS) Group. Effect of intensive blood-glucose control with metformin on complications in overweight patients with type 2 diabetes (UKPDS 34). Lancet 1998;352:854–865.

153. UK Prospective Diabetes Study (UKPDS) Group. Intensive blood-glucose control with sulphonylureas or insulin compared with conventional treatment and risk of complications in patients with type 2 diabetes (UKPDS 33). Lancet 1998;352:837–853.

154. Fullert S, Schneir F, Haak E, et al. Effects of pioglitazone in nondiabetic patients with arterial hypertension: a double-blind, placebo-controlled study. J Clin Endocrinol Metab 2002;87(12):5503–5506.

155. Pfutzner A, Marx N, Lubben G, et al. Improvement of cardiovascular risk markers by pioglitazone is independent from glycemic control: results from the pioneer study. J Am Coll Cardiol 2005;45(12):1925–1931.

156. Dormandy JA, Charbonnel B, Eckland DJ, et al; PROactive investigators. Secondary prevention of macrovascular events in patients with type 2 diabetes in the PROactive Study (PROspective pioglitAzone Clinical Trial In macroVascular Events): a randomised controlled trial. Lancet 2005;366:1279-1289.

157. Freemantle N. How well does the evidence on pioglitazone back up researchers' claims for a reduction in macrovascular events? BMJ 2005;331:836-838.

158. Van Wijk JP, de Koning EJ, Castro Cabezas M, Rabelink TJ. Rosiglitazone improves postprandial triglyceride and free fatty acid metabolism in type 2 diabetes. Diabetes Care 2005;28(4):844–849.

159. Raji A, Seely EW, Bekins SA, et al. Rosiglitazone improves insulin sensitivity and lowers blood pressure in hypertensive patients. Diabetes Care 2003;26(1):172–178.

160. Derosa G, Cicero AF, Gaddi A, et al. Metabolic effects of pioglitazone and rosiglitazone in patients with diabetes and metabolic syndrome treated with glimepiride: a twelve-month, multicenter, double-blind, randomized, controlled, parallel-group trial. Clin Ther 2004;26(5):744–754.

161. Home PD, Pocock SJ, Beck-Nielsen H, et al. Rosiglitazone evaluated for cardiac outcomes and regulation of glycaemia in diabetes (RECORD): study design and protocol. Diabetologia 2005;48(9):1726–1735.

162. Hubacek J, Verma S, Shewchuk L, et al. Rationale and design of the glitazones and the endothelium (GATE) study: evaluation of rosiglitazone on endothelial function in patients with diabetes. Can J Cardiol 2004;20(14):1449–1453.

163. Nissen SE, Wolski K, Topol EJ. Effect of muraglitazar on death and major adverse cardiovascular events in patients with type 2 diabetes mellitus. JAMA 2005;294(20):2581–2586.

164. Gautier JF, Fetita S, Sobngwi E, Salaün-Martin C. Biological actions of the incretins GIP and GLP-1 and therapeutic perspectives in patients with type 2 diabetes. Diabetes Metab 2005;31:233–242.

165. Holst JJ. Glucagon-like peptide-1: from extract to agent. The Claude Bernard Lecture, 2005. Diabetologia 2006;49:253–260.

166. Diabetes UK. Recommendations for the Management of Diabetes in Primary Care, 2nd edition. London: Diabetes UK, 2000.

167. Ahn CW, Song YD, Kim JH, et al. The validity of random urine specimen albumin measurement as a screening test for diabetic nephropathy. Yonsei Med J 1999;40:40–45.

168. Damsgaard EM, Froland A, Jorgensen OD, Mogensen CE. Eight to nine year mortality in known non-insulin dependent diabetics and controls. Kidney Int 1992;41:731–735.

169. Brancati FL, Whelton PK, Randall BL, et al. Risk of end-stage renal disease in diabetes mellitus: a prospective cohort study of men screened for MRFIT. Multiple Risk Factor Intervention Trial. JAMA 1997;278:2069–2074.

170. Eastman RC, Keen H. The impact of cardiovascular disease on people with diabetes: the potential for prevention. Lancet 1997;350(suppl 1):S129–S132.

171. Kuusisto J, Mykkanen L, Pyorala K, Laakso M. Hyperinsulinemic microalbuminuria. A new risk indicator for coronary heart disease. Circulation 1995;91:831–837.

172. Mogensen CE, Poulsen PL. Epidemiology of microalbuminuria in diabetes and in the background population. Curr Opin Nephrol Hypertens 1994;3:248–256.

173. Conlon PJ, Kovalik E, Schumm D, et al. Normalization of hematocrit in hemodialysis patients with cardiac disease does not increase blood pressure. Ren Fail 2000;22:435–444.

174. Mogensen CE, Petersen MM, Hansen KW, Christensen CK. Micro-albuminuria and the organ-damage concept in antihypertensive therapy for patients with insulin-dependent diabetes mellitus. J Hypertens 1992;10(suppl):S43–S51.

175. Mogensen CE. Microalbuminuria, blood pressure and diabetic renal disease: origin and development of ideas. Diabetologia 1999;42:263–285.

176. Ewald B, Attia J. Which test to detect microalbuminuria in diabetic patients? A systematic review. Aust Fam Physician 2004;33:565–677.

177. American Diabetes Association. Clinical practice recommendations 2000. Diabetes Care 2000;23(suppl 1):S1–S116.

178. Hansson L, Hedner T, Himmelmann A. The 1999 WHO-ISH guidelines for the management of hypertension – new targets, new treatment and a comprehensive approach to total cardiovascular risk reduction. Blood Press 1999;(suppl 1):3–5.

179. Feldman RD. The 1999 Canadian recommendations for the management of hypertension. On behalf of the Task Force for the Development of the 1999 Canadian Recommendations for the Management of Hypertension. Can J Cardiol 1999;15(suppl G):57G–64G.

180. Bakris GL, Williams M, Dworkin L, et al. Preserving renal function in adults with hypertension and diabetes: a consensus approach. National Kidney Foundation Hypertension and Diabetes Executive Committees Working Group. Am J Kid Dis 2000;36:646–661.

181. Mogensen CE, Chachati A, Christensen CK, et al. Microalbuminuria: an early marker of renal involvement in diabetes. Uremia Invest 1985;9:85–95.

182. Ruilope LM, Salvetti A, Jamerson K, et al. Renal function and intensive lowering of blood pressure in hypertensive participants of the hypertension optimal treatment (HOT) study. J Am Soc Nephrol 2001;12:218–225.

183. Marre M, Lievre M, Vasmant D, et al. Determinants of elevated urinary albumin in the 4,937 type 2 diabetic subjects recruited for the DIABHYCAR Study in Western Europe and North Africa. Diabetes Care 2000;23(suppl 2):B40–B48.

184. Ravid M, Brosh D, Ravid-Safran D, et al. Main risk factors for nephropathy in type 2 diabetes mellitus are plasma cholesterol levels, mean blood pressure, and hyperglycemia. Arch Int Med 1998;158:998–1004.

185. Nielsen S, Schmitz A, Poulsen PL, et al. Albuminuria and 24-h ambulatory blood pressure in normoalbuminuric and microalbuminuric NIDDM patients. A longitudinal study. Diabetes Care 1995;18:1434–1441.

186. Mathiesen ER, Hommel E, Hansen HP, et al. Randomised controlled trial of long term efficacy of captopril on preservation of kidney function in normotensive patients with insulin dependent diabetes and microalbuminuria. BMJ 1999;319:24–25.

187. Rossing P, Hommel E, Smidt UM, Parving HH. Reduction in albuminuria predicts a beneficial effect on diminishing the progression of human diabetic nephropathy during antihypertensive treatment. Diabetologia 1994;37:511–516.

188. The EUCLID Study Group. Randomised placebo-controlled trial of lisinopril in normotensive patients with insulin-dependent diabetes and normoalbuminuria or microalbuminuria. Lancet 1997;349:1787–1792.

189. Heart Outcomes Prevention Evaluation Study Investigators. Effects of ramipril on cardiovascular and microvascular outcomes in people with diabetes mellitus: results of the HOPE study and MICRO-HOPE substudy. Lancet 2000;355:253–259.

190. Laffel LM, McGill JB, Gans DJ. The beneficial effect of angiotensin-converting enzyme inhibition with captopril on diabetic nephropathy in normotensive IDDM patients with microalbuminuria. North American Microalbuminuria Study Group. Am J Med 1995;99:497–504.

191. Ravid M, Savin H, Jutrin I, et al. Long-term stabilizing effect of angiotensin-converting enzyme inhibition on plasma creatinine and on proteinuria in normotensive type II diabetic patients. Ann Intern Med 1993;118:577–581.

192. Sano T, Hotta N, Kawamura T, et al. Effects of long-term enalapril treatment on persistent microalbuminuria in normotensive type 2 diabetic patients: results of a 4-year, prospective, randomised study. Diabet Med 1996;13:120–124.

193. Estacio RO, Jeffers BW, Gifford N, Schrier RW. Effect of blood pressure control on diabetic microvascular complications in patients with hypertension and type 2 diabetes. Diabetes Care 2000;23(suppl 2):B54–B64.

194. Schnack C, Hoffmann W, Hopmeier P, Schernthaner G. Renal and metabolic effects of 1-year treatment with ramipril or atenolol in NIDDM patients with microalbuminuria. Diabetologia 1996;39:1611–1616.

195. Capek M, Schnack C, Ludvik B, et al. Effects of captopril treatment versus placebo on renal function in type 2 diabetic patients with microalbuminuria: a long-term study. Clin Investig 1994;72:961–966.

196. Lebovitz HE, Wiegmann TB, Cnaan A, et al. Renal protective effects of enalapril in hypertensive NIDDM: role of baseline albuminuria. Kidney Int 1994;45(suppl):S150–S155.

197. Trevisan R, Tiengo A. Effect of low-dose ramipril on microalbuminuria in normotensive or mild hypertensive non-insulin-dependent diabetic patients. Am J Hypertens 1995;8:876–883.

198. Parving HH, Lehnert H, Brochner-Mortensen J, et al. The effect of irbesartan on the development of diabetic nephropathy in patients with type 2 diabetes. N Engl J Med 2001;345:870–878.

199. Mathiesen ER, Hommel E, Giese J, Parving HH. Efficacy of captopril in postponing nephropathy in normotensive insulin dependent diabetic patients with microalbuminuria. BMJ 1991;303:81–87.

200. Teo K, Yusuf S, Sleight P, et al; for the ONTARGET/TRANSCEND Investigators. Rationale, design, and baseline characteristics of 2 large, simple, randomised trials evaluating telmisartan, ramipril, and their combination in high-risk patients: the Ongoing Telmisartan Alone and in Combination with Ramipril Global Endpoint Trial/Telmisartan Randomised Assessment Study in ACE Intolerant Subjects with Cardiovascular Disease (ONTARGET/TRANSCEND) trials. Am Heart J 2004;148:52–61.

201. Bakris GL, Copley JB, Vicknair N, Sadler R, Leurgans S. Calcium channel blockers versus other antihypertensive therapies on progression of NIDDM associated nephropathy. Kidney Int 1996;50:1641–1650.

202. Hansson L, Zanchetti A, Carruthers SG, et al. Effects of intensive blood-pressure lowering and low-dose aspirin in patients with hypertension: principal results of the Hypertension Optimal Treatment (HOT) randomised trial. HOT Study Group. Lancet 1998;351:1755–1762.

203. Tuomilehto J, Rastenyte D, Birkenhager WH, et al. Effects of calcium-channel blockade in older patients with diabetes and systolic hypertension. Systolic Hypertension in Europe Trial Investigators. N Engl J Med 1999;340:677–684.

204. Birkenhager WH, Staessen JA, Gasowski J, de Leeuw PW. Effects of antihypertensive treatment on endpoints in the diabetic patients randomised in the Systolic Hypertension in Europe (Syst-Eur) trial. J Nephrol 2000;13:232–237.

205. Bakris GL, Mangrum A, Copley JB, et al. Effect of calcium channel or beta-blockade on the progression of diabetic nephropathy in African Americans. Hypertension 1997;29:744–750.

206. Fogari R, Corradi L, Poletti L, et al. Effects of fosinopril amlodipine combination on microalbuminuria in hypertensive patietns with type 2 diabetes. Am J Hypertens 2000;13:K023.

207. Bakris G, White D. Effects of an ACE inhibitor combined with a calcium channel blocker on progression of diabetic nephropathy. J Hum Hypertens 1997;11:35–38.

208. Mogensen CE, Neldam S, Tikkanen I, et al. Randomised controlled trial of dual blockade of renin-angiotensin system in patients with hypertension, microalbuminuria, and non-insulin dependent diabetes: the candesartan and lisinopril microalbuminuria (CALM) study. BMJ 2000;321:1440–1444.

209. Krolewski AS, Laffel LM, Krolewski M, et al. Glycosylated hemoglobin and the risk of microalbuminuria in patients with insulin-dependent diabetes mellitus. N Engl J Med 1995;332:1251–1255.

210. Warram JH, Gearin G, Laffel L, Krolewski AS. Effect of duration of type I diabetes on the prevalence of stages of diabetic nephropathy defined by urinary albumin/creatinine ratio. J Am Soc Nephrol 1996;7:930–937.

211. Nielsen S, Schmitz A, Rehling M, Mogensen CE. The clinical course of renal function in NIDDM patients with normo- and microalbuminuria. J Intern Med 1997;241:133–141.

212. Bennett PH, Haffner S, Kasiske BL, et al. Screening and management of microalbuminuria in patients with diabetes mellitus: recommendations to the Scientific Advisory Board of the National Kidney Foundation from an ad hoc committee of the Council on Diabetes Mellitus of the National Kidney Foundation. Am J Kidney Dis 1995;25:107–112.

213. Krolewski AS, Warram JH, Christlieb AR, et al. The changing natural history of nephropathy in type I diabetes. Am J Med 1985;78:785–794.

214. Parving HH. Is antihypertensive treatment the same for NIDDM and IDDM patients? Diabetes Res Clin Prac 1998;39(suppl):S43–S47.

215. Myers BD, Nelson RG, Tan M, et al. Progression of overt nephropathy in non-insulin-dependent diabetes. Kidney Int 1995;47:1781–1789.

216. Berrut G, Bouhanick B, Fabbri P, et al. Microalbuminuria as a predictor of a drop in glomerular filtration rate in subjects with non-insulin-dependent diabetes mellitus and hypertension. Clin Nephrol 1997;48:92–97.

217. Andersen S, Blouch K, Bialek J, et al. Glomerular permselectivity in early stages of overt diabetic nephropathy. Kidney Int 2000;58:2129–2137.

218. Lemley KV, Abdullah I, Myers BD, et al. Evolution of incipient nephropathy in type 2 diabetes mellitus. Kidney Int 2000;58:1228–1237.
219. Warram JH, Sigal RJ, Martin BC, et al. Natural history of impaired glucose tolerance: follow-up at Joslin Clinic. Diabet Med 1996;13:S40–S45.
220. Krolewski M, Eggers PW, Warram JH. Magnitude of end-stage renal disease in IDDM: a 35 year follow-up study. Kidney Int 1996;50:2041–2046.
221. Krolewski AS, Warram JH, Freire MB. Epidemiology of late diabetic complications. A basis for the development and evaluation of preventive programs. Endocrin Metab Clinics North Am 1996;25:217–242.
222. Parving HH, Andersen AR, Smidt UM, et al. Effect of antihypertensive treatment on kidney function in diabetic nephropathy. BMJ Clin Res 1987;294:1443–1447.
223. United States Renal Data System. Causes of death. Am J Kid Dis 1998;32(suppl):S81–S88.
224. Kasiske BL, Lakatua JD, Ma JZ, Louis TA. A meta-analysis of the effects of dietary protein restriction on the rate of decline in renal function. Am J Kidney Dis 1998;31:954–961.
225. Lewis EJ, Hunsicker LG, Bain RP, Rohde RD. The effect of angiotensin-converting-enzyme inhibition on diabetic nephropathy. The collaborative study group. N Engl J Med 1993;329:1456–1462.
226. Cooper ME. Renal protection and angiotensin converting enzyme inhibition in microalbuminuric type I and type II diabetic patients. J Hypertens 1996;14(suppl):S11–S14.
227. Tatti P, Pahor M, Byington RP, et al. Outcome results of the Fosinopril Versus Amlodipine Cardiovascular Events Randomised Trial (FACET) in patients with hypertension and NIDDM. Diabetes Care 1998;21:597–603.
228. Estacio RO, Jeffers BW, Hiatt WR, et al. The effect of nisoldipine as compared with enalapril on cardiovascular outcomes in patients with non-insulin-dependent diabetes and hypertension. N Engl J Med 1998;338:645–652.
229. Agodoa LY, Appel L, Bakris GL, et al. Effect of ramipril vs amlodipine on renal outcomes in hypertensive nephrosclerosis: a randomized controlled trial. JAMA 2001;285:2719–2728.
230. Pahor M, Psaty BM, Alderman MH, et al. Health outcomes associated with calcium antagonists compared with other first-line antihypertensive therapies: a meta-analysis of randomised controlled trials. Lancet 2000;356:1949–1954.
231. Lewis EJ, Hunsicker LG, Clarke WR, et al. Renoprotective effect of the angiotensin-receptor antagonist irbesartan in patients with nephropathy due to type 2 diabetes. N Engl J Med 2001;345:851–860.
232. Binik YM, Devins GM, Barre PE, et al. Live and learn: patient education delays the need to initiate renal replacement therapy in end-stage renal disease. J Nerv Ment Dis 1993;181:371–376.
233. Christensen PK, Rossing P, Nielsen FS, Parving HH. Natural course of kidney function in Type 2 diabetic patients with diabetic nephropathy. Diabet Med 1999;16:388–394.
234. Frick MH, Elo O, Haapa K, et al. Helsinki Heart Study: primary-prevention trial with gemfibrozil in middle-aged men with dyslipidemia–safety of treatment, changes in risk factors, and incidence of coronary heart disease. N Engl J Med 1987;317:1237–1245.
235. Committee of Principal Investigators. A co-operative trial in the primary prevention of ischemic heart disease using clofibrate: report from the Committee of Principal Investigators. Br Heart J 1978;40:1069–1118.
236. Lipid Research Clinics Program. The Lipid Research Clinics Coronary Primary Prevention Trial results, I: reduction in incidence of coronary heart disease. JAMA 1984;251:351–364.
237. Law MR, Wald NJ, Thompson SG. By how much and how quickly does reduction in serum cholesterol concentration lower risk of ischemic heart disease? BMJ 1994;308:367–373.
238. Serruys PW, de Feyter P, Macaya C, et al; Intervention Prevention Study (LIPS) Investigators. Fluvastatin for prevention of cardiac events following successful first percutaneous coronary intervention: a randomised controlled trial. JAMA 2002;287:3215–3222.
239. Shepherd J, Cobbe SM, Ford I, et al; for the West of Scotland Coronary Prevention Study Group. Prevention of coronary heart disease with pravastatin in men with hypercholesterolemia. N Engl J Med 1995;333:1301–1307.
240. Buchwald H, Varco RL, Matts JP, et al. Report of the program on the surgical control of the hyperlipidemias (POSCH): effect of partial ileal bypass surgery on mortality and morbidity from coronary heart disease in patients with hypercholesterolemia. N Engl J Med 1990;323:946–955.
241. Rubins HB, Robins SJ, Collins D, et al; for the Veterans Affairs High-Density Lipoprotein Cholesterol Intervention Trial Study Group. Gemfibrozil for the secondary prevention of coronary heart disease in men with low levels of high-density lipoprotein cholesterol. N Engl J Med 1999;341:410–418.
242. Eastern Stroke and Coronary Heart Disease Collaborative Research Group. Blood pressure, cholesterol, and stroke in eastern Asia. Lancet 1998;352:1801–1807.
243. Tanne D, Koren-Morag N, Graff E, Goldbourt U. Blood lipids and first-ever ischemic stroke/transient ischemic attack in the Bezafibrate Infarction Prevention (BIP) Registry: high triglycerides constitute an independent risk factor. Circulation 2001;104:2892–2897.
244. Crouse JR III, Byington RP, Furberg CD. HMG-CoA reductase inhibitor therapy and stroke risk reduction: an analysis of clinical trials data. Atherosclerosis 1998;138:11–24.
245. Bucher HC, Griffith LE, Guyatt GH. Systematic review on the risk and benefit of different cholesterol-lowering interventions. Arterioscler Thromb Vasc Biol 1999;19:187–195.
246. Kannel WB, Thomas HE, Kjelsberg MO. Overall and coronary heart disease mortality rates in relation to major risk factors in 325,348 men screened for the MRFIT. Am Heart J 1986;112:825–836.
247. SHEP Co-operative Research Group. Prevention of stroke by antihypertensive drug treatment in older persons with isolated systolic hypertension: final results of the Systolic Hypertension in the Elderly Program (SHEP). JAMA 1991;265:3255–3264.

143

248. Zemel PC, Sowers JR. Relation between lipids and atherosclerosis: epidemiologic evidence and clinical implications. Am J Cardiol 1990;66:7i–12i.
249. Primatesta P, Poulter NR. Lipid levels and the use of lipid-lowering agents in England and Scotland. Eur J Cardiovasc Prev Rehabil 2004;11:484–488.
250. Heart and Stroke Foundation of Canada. The growing burden of heart disease and stroke in Canada 2003. May 2003.
251. Schwartz GG, Olsson AG, Ezekowitz MD, et al. Effects of atorvastatin on early recurrent ischemic events in acute coronary syndromes. JAMA 2001;285:1711–1718.
252. Martin MJ, Hulley SB, Browner WS, et al. Serum cholesterol, blood pressure and mortality: implications from a cohort of 361,662 men. Lancet 1986;2:933–936.
253. Yusuf S, Anand S. Cost of prevention. The case of lipid lowering. Circulation 1996;93:1774–1776.
254. Maron DJ, Fazio S, Linton MF. Current perspectives on statins. Circulation 2000;18:207–213.
255. West of Scotland Coronary Prevention Study. Identification of high-risk groups and comparison with other cardiovascular intervention trials. Lancet 1996;348:1339–1342.
256. Hazzard WR, Ettinger WH Jr. The effect of pravastatin on coronary events after myocardial infarction. N Engl J Med 1997;336:961.
257. Miller M, Bachorik PS, McCrindle BW, Kwiterovich PO Jr. Effect of gemfibrozil in men with primary isolated low high-density lipoprotein cholesterol: a randomised, double-blind, placebo-controlled, crossover study. Am J Med 1993;94:7–12.
258. Bloomfield Rubins H, Davenport J, Babikian V, et al; VA-HIT Study Group. Reduction in stroke with gemfibrozil in men with coronary heart disease and low HDL cholesterol: The Veterans Affairs HDL Intervention Trial (VA-HIT). Circulation 2001;103:2828–2833.
259. Haffner SM. Coronary heart disease in patients with diabetes. N Engl J Med 2000;342:1040–1042.
260. Effect of fenofibrate on progression of coronary-artery disease in type 2 diabetes: the Diabetes Atherosclerosis Intervention Study, a randomised study. Lancet 2001;357:905–910.
261. Freeman DJ, Norrie J, Sattar N, et al. Pravastatin and the development of diabetes mellitus: evidence for a protective treatment effect in the West of Scotland Coronary Prevention Study. Circulation 2001;103:357–362.
262. Haq IU, Wallis EJ, Jackson PR, et al. Implication of recent trials with b-hydroxy-b-methylglutaryl coenzyme A reductase inhibitors for hypertension management. J Hypertens 1999;17:1641–1646.
263. Green R, Kwok S, Durrington PN. Preventing cardiovascular disease in hypertension: effects of lowering blood pressure and cholesterol. QJM 2002;95:821–826.
264. Hebert PR, Gaziano JM, Chan KS, Hennekens CH. Cholesterol lowering with statin drugs, risk of stroke, and total mortality. An overview of randomized trials. JAMA 1997;278:313–321.
265. Collins R, MacMahon S. Blood pressure, antihypertensive drug treatment and the risks of stroke and of coronary heart disease. Br Med Bull 1994;50:272–298.
266. Amarenco P, Tonkin AM. Statins for stroke prevention: disappointment and hope. Circulation 2004;109(suppl 1):44–49.
267. Samuelsson O, Wilhelmsen L, Andersson OK, et al. Cardiovascular morbidity in relation to change in blood pressure and serum cholesterol levels in treated hypertension: results from the primary prevention trial in Goteborg, Sweden. JAMA 1987;258:1768–1776.
268. The ALLHAT Officers and Coordinators for the ALLHAT Collaborative Research Group. Major outcomes in moderately hypercholesterolemic, hypertensive patients randomised to pravastatin vs usual care; the Antihypertensive and Lipid-Lowering Treatment to Prevent Heart Attack Trial (ALLHAT-LLT). JAMA 2002;288:2998–3007.
269. The ALLHAT Officers and Coordinators for the ALLHAT Collaborative Research Group. Major outcomes in high-risk hypertensive patients randomised to angiotensin-converting enzyme inhibitor or calcium channel blocker vs diuretic: the Antihypertensive and Lipid-Lowering Treatment to Prevent Heart Attack Trial (ALLHAT). JAMA 2002;288:2981–2997.
270. Sever PS, Dahlöf B, Poulter NR, et al. Rationale, design, methods and baseline demography of participants of the Anglo-Scandinavian Cardiac Outcomes Trial. J Hypertens 2001;6:1139–1147.
271. Sever PS, Dahlöf B, Poulter NR, et al. Prevention of coronary and stroke events with atorvastatin in hypertensive patients who have average or lower-than-average cholesterol concentrations, in the Anglo-Scandinavian Cardiac Outcomes Trial–Lipid Lowering Arm (ASCOT-LLA): a multicentre randomised controlled trial. Lancet 2003;361:1149–1158.
272. Ramsay LE, Williams B, Johnston GD, et al. Guidelines for management of hypertension: report of the third working party of the British Hypertension Society. J Hum Hypertens 1999;13:569–592.
273. O'Callaghan CJ, Krum H, Conway EL, et al. Short term effects of pravastatin on blood pressure in hypercholesterolaemic hypertensive patients. Blood Press 1994;3:404–406.
274. Straznicky NE, Howes LG, Lam W, Louis WJ. Effects of pravastatin on cardiovascular reactivity to norepinephrine and angiotensin II in patients with hypercholesterolemia and systemic hypertension. Am J Cardiol 1995;75:582–586.
275. Glorioso N, Troffa C, Filigheddu F, et al. Effect of the HMG-CoA reductase inhibitors on blood pressure in patients with essential hypertension and primary hypercholesterolemia. Hypertension 1999;34:1281–1286.
276. Ferrier KE, Muhlmann MH, Baguet JP, et al. Intensive cholesterol reduction lowers blood pressure and large artery stiffness in isolated systolic hypertension. J Am Coll Cardiol 2002;39:1020–1025.
277. EUROASPIRE II Study Group. Lifestyle and risk factor management and use of drug therapies in coronary patients from 15 countries. Eur Heart J 2001;22:554–572.

278. Forette F, Seux ML, Staessen JA, et al. Prevention of dementia in randomised double-blind placebo-controlled systolic hypertension in Europe (Syst-Eur) trial. Lancet 1998;352:1347–1351.

279. Clarke CE. Does the treatment of isolated systolic hypertension prevent dementia? J Hum Hypertens 1999;13:357–358.

280. Khan N, Campbell NRC. Lack of control of high blood pressure and treatment recommendations in Canada. Can J Cardiol 2002;18:657–661.

281. Neaton JD, Wentworth D. Serum cholesterol, blood pressure, cigarette smoking, and death from coronary heart disease. Overall findings and differences by age for 316,099 white men. Multiple Risk Factor Intervention Trial Research group. Arch Intern Med 1992;152:56–64.

282. Lloyd A, Schmieder C, Marchant N. Financial and health costs of uncontrolled blood pressure in the United Kingdom. Pharmacoeconomics 2003;21(suppl 1):33–41.

283. Chobanian AV, Bakris GL, Black HR, et al. National Heart, Lung, and Blood Institute Joint National Committee on Prevention, Detection, Evaluation, and Treatment of High Blood Pressure; National High Blood Pressure Education Program Coordinating Committee. The Seventh Report of the Joint National Committee on Prevention, Detection, Evaluation, and Treatment of High Blood Pressure: the JNC 7 report. JAMA 2003;289:2560–2572.

284. O'Rourke M, Frohlich ED. Pulse pressure. Is this a clinically useful risk factor? Hypertension 1999;34:372–374.

285. Domanski MJ, Davis BR, Pfeiffer MA, et al. Isolated systolic hypertension. Prognostic information provided by pulse pressure. Hypertension 1999;34:375–380.

286. Kannel WB. Elevated systolic blood pressure as a cardiovascular risk factor. Am J Cardiol 2000;85:251–255.

287. Whelton PK, He J, Muntner P. Prevalence, awareness, treatment and control of hypertension in North America, North Africa and Asia. J Hum Hypertens 2004;18:545–551.

288. Joffres MR, Ghadirian P, Fodor JG, et al. Awareness, treatment, and control of hypertension in Canada. Am J Hypertens 1997;10:1097–1102.

289. Rutan G, Kuller LH, Neaton JD, et al. Mortality associated with diastolic hypertension and isolated systolic hypertension among men screened for the Multiple Risk Factor Intervention Trial. Circulation 1988;77:504–514.

290. Franklin SS, Khan SA, Wong ND, et al. Is pulse pressure useful in predicting risk for coronary heart disease? The Framingham Heart Study. Circulation 1999;100:354–360.

291. Campbell NRC, Chockalingam A, Fodor JG, et al. Errors in assessment of blood pressure. Blood pressure measuring technique. Can J Pub Health 1994;85:18s–21s.

292. European Society of Hypertension–European Society of Cardiology Guidelines Committee. 2003 European Society of Hypertension–European Society of Cardiology guidelines for the management of arterial hypertension. J Hypertens 2003;21:1011–1053.

293. Campbell NR, McKay DW, Chockalingam A, et al. Errors in assessment of blood pressure: sphygmomanometers and blood pressure cuffs. Can J Pub Health 1994;85:22s–25s.

294. Palatini P. Limitations of ambulatory blood pressure monitoring. Blood Press Monit 2001;6:221–224.

295. Palatini P, Dorigatti F, Roman E, et al. White-coat hypertension: a selection bias? J Hypertens 1998;16:977–984.

296. Johnson AL, Taylor DW, Sacket DL. Self-recording of blood pressure in the management of hypertension. CMAJ 1978;119:1034–1039.

297. O'Brien E, Petrie J, Littler WA, et al. The British Hypertension Society Protocol for the evaluation of blood pressure measuring devices. J Hypertens 1993;11(suppl 2):S43–S63.

298. American National Standard. Electronic or Automated Sphygmomanometers. ANSI/AAMI SP10-1992. Arlington VA, USA: Association for the Advancement of Medical Instrumentation, 1993; pp. 40.

299. Pickering T. Recommendations for the use of home (self) and ambulatory blood pressure monitoring. Am J Hypertens 1995;9:1–11.

300. O'Brien E, Asmar R, Beilin L, et al; European Society of Hypertension Working Group on Blood Pressure Monitoring. Practice guidelines of the European Society of Hypertension for clinic, ambulatory and self blood pressure measurement. J Hypertens 2005;23:697–701.

301. Omboni S, Parati G, Palatini P, et al. Reproducibility and clinical value of nocturnal hypotension: prospective evidence from the SAMPLE study. J Hypertens 1998;16:733–738.

302. Wilkinson IB, Franklin SS, Cockcroft JR. Nitric oxide and the regulation of large artery stiffness: from physiology to pharmacology. Hypertension 2004;44:112–116.

303. Cockcroft JR, Wilkinson IB. Arterial stiffness and pulse contour analysis: an age old concept revisited. Clin Sci 2002;103:379–380.

304. Montgomery AA, Fahey T, Peters TJ, et al. Evaluation of computer based clinical decision support system and risk chart for management of hypertension in primary care: randomised controlled trial. BMJ 2000;329:686–690.

305. MacMahon S, Peto R, Cutler J, et al. Blood pressure, stroke, and coronary heart disease. Part 1. Prolonged differences in blood pressure: prospective observational studies corrected for the regression dilution bias. Lancet 1990;335:765–774.

306. Collins R, Peto R, MacMahon S, et al. Blood pressure, stroke, and coronary heart disease. Part 2. Short-term reductions in blood pressure: overview of randomised drug trials and their epidemiological context. Lancet 1990;335:827–838.

307. He J, Whelton PK. Elevated systolic blood pressure and risk of cardiovascular and renal disease: overview of evidence from observational epidemiologic studies and randomised controlled trials. Am Heart J 1999;138:211–219.

308. Wing LMH, Reid CM, Ryan P, et al. A comparison of outcomes with angiotensin-converting-enzyme inhibitors and diuretics for hypertension in the elderly. N Engl J Med 2003;348:583–592.

309. Brown MJ, Palmer CT, Castaigne A, et al. Morbidity and mortality in patients randomised to double-blind treatment with a long-acting calcium-channel blocker or diuretic in the International Nifedipine GITS Study: Intervention as a Goal in Hypertension Treatment (INSIGHT). Lancet 2000;356:366–372.

310. Dahlof B, Devereux RB, Kjeldsen SE, et al. Cardiovascular morbidity and mortality in the Losartan Intervention For Endpoint Reduction in hypertension study (LIFE): a randomised trial against atenolol. Lancet 2002;359:995–1003.

311. Dahlof B, Lindholm LH, Hansson L, et al. Morbidity and mortality in the Swedish Trial in Old Patients with Hypertension (STOP-Hypertension). Lancet 1991;338:1281–1285.

312. Julius S, Kjeldsen S, Weber M, et al. Outcomes in hypertensive patients at high cardiovascular risk treated with regimens based on valsartan or amlodipine: the VALUE randomised trial. Lancet 2004;363:2022–2031.

313. Dahlof B, Sever PS, Poulter NR, et al; ASCOT Investigators. Prevention of cardiovascular events with an antihypertensive regimen of amlodipine adding perindopril as required versus atenolol adding bendroflumethiazide as required, in the Anglo-Scandinavian Cardiac Outcomes Trial-Blood Pressure Lowering Arm (ASCOT-BPLA): a multicentre randomised controlled trial. Lancet 2005;366:895–906.

314. Staessen J, Wang J, Birkenhager W. Outcome beyond blood pressure control? Eur Heart J 2003;24:504–514.

315. Lindholm LH, Ibsen H, Borch-Johnsen K, et al; for the LIFE study group. Risk of new-onset diabetes in the Losartan Intervention For Endpoint reduction in hypertension study. J Hypertens 2002;20:1879–1886.

316. Weber MA, Julius S, Kjeldsen SE, et al. Blood pressure dependent and independent effects of antihypertensive treatment on clinical events in the VALUE Trial. Lancet 2004;363:2049–2051.

317. Yusuf S, Sleight P, Pogue J, et al. Effects of an angiotensin-converting-enzyme inhibitor, ramipril, on cardiovascular events in high-risk patients. The Heart Outcomes Prevention Evaluation Study Investigators. N Engl J Med 2000;342:145–153.

318. Fox KM; EURopean trial On reduction of cardiac events with Perindopril in stable coronary Artery disease investigators. Efficacy of perindopril in reduction of cardiovascular events among patients with stable coronary disease: randomised, double-blind, placebo-controlled, multicentre trial (the EUROPA study). Lancet 2003;362:782–788.

319. Furberg CD, Psaty BM, Meyer JV. Nifedipine: dose-related increase in mortality in patients with coronary heart disease. Circulation 1995;92:1326–1331.

320. Opie LH, Schall R. Evidence-based evaluation of calcium channel blockers for hypertension. J Am Coll Cardiol 2002;39:315–322.

321. Blood Pressure Lowering Treatment Trialists' Collaboration. Effects of ACE inhibitors, calcium antagonists, and other blood pressure lowering drugs: results of prospectively designed overviews of randomised trials. Lancet 2000;356:1955–1964.

322. Neaton JD, Grimm RH Jr, Prineas RJ, et al. Treatment of mild hypertension study. Final results. JAMA 1993;270:713–724.

323. Grimm RH, Grandits GA, Prineas RJ, et al. Long-term effects on sexual function of five antihypertensive drugs and nutritional hygienic treatment in hypertensive men and women. Treatment of Mild Hypertension Study (TOMHS). Hypertension 1997;29:8–14.

324. Cushman WC, Khatri I, Materson BJ, et al. Treatment of hypertension in the elderly. III. Response of isolated systolic hypertension to various doses of hydrochlorothiazide: results of a Department of Veterans Affairs cooperative study. Department of Veterans Affairs Cooperative Study Group on Antihypertensive Agents. Arch Intern Med 1991;151:1954–1960.

325. Savage PJ, Pressel SL, Curb JD, et al. Influence of long-term, low-dose, diuretic-based, antihypertensive therapy on glucose, lipid, uric acid, and potassium levels in older men and women with isolated systolic hypertension: the systolic hypertension in the elderly program. SHEP Cooperative Research Group. Arch Intern Med 1998;158:741–751.

326. Applegate WB, Pressel S, Wittes J, et al. Impact of the treatment of isolated systolic hypertension on behavioral variables. Results from the systolic hypertension in the elderly program. Arch Intern Med 1994;154:2154–2160.

327. Franse LV, Pahor M, Di Bari M, et al. Hypokalemia associated with diuretic use and cardiovascular events in the Systolic Hypertension in the Elderly Program. Hypertension 2000;35:1025–1030.

328. Materson BJ, Reda DJ, Cushman WC, et al. Single-drug therapy for hypertension in men. A comparison of six antihypertensive agents with placebo. N Engl J Med 1993;328:914–921.

329. Murdoch D, Heel RC. Amlodipine. A review of its pharmacodynamic and pharmacokinetic properties, and therapeutic use in cardiovascular disease. Drugs 1991;41:478–505.

330. Saltiel E, Ellrodt AG, Monk JP, et al. Felodipine. A review of its pharmacodynamic and pharmacokinetic properties, and therapeutic use in hypertension. Drugs 1988;36:387–428.

331. Medical Research Council Working Party. Medical Research Council trial of treatment of hypertension in older adults: principal results. BMJ 1992;304:405–412.

332. Bakris GL, Fonseca V, Katholi RE, et al; GEMINI Investigators. Metabolic effects of carvedilol vs metoprolol in patients with type 2 diabetes mellitus and hypertension: a randomized controlled trial. JAMA 2004;292(18):2227–2236.

333. Brown MJ, Cruickshank JK, Dominiczak AF, et al. Better blood pressure control: how to combine drugs. J Hum Hypertens 2003;17:81–86.

334. Dickerson JEC, Hingorani AD, Ashby MJ, et al. Optimisation of antihypertensive treatment by crossover rotation of four major classes. Lancet 1999;353:2008–2013.

335. Jones JK, Gorkin L, Lian JF, et al. Discontinuation of and changes in treatment after start of new courses of antihypertensive drugs: a study of a United Kingdom population. BMJ 1995;311:293–295.

336. Gueyffier F, Bulpitt C, Boissel J-P. Antihypertensive drugs in very old people: a subgroup meta-analysis of randomised controlled trials. Lancet 1999;353:793–796.
337. Walker WG, Hermann J, Murphy R, Patz A. Elevated blood pressure and angiotensin II are associated with accelerated loss of renal function in diabetic nephropathy. Trans Am Clin Climatol Assoc 1985;97:94–104.
338. Schiffrin EL. Vascular protection with newer antihypertensive agents. J Hypertens 1998;16(suppl):S25–S29.
339. Hansson L, Lindholm LH, Niskanen L, et al. Effect of angiotensin-converting-enzyme inhibition compared with conventional therapy on cardiovascular morbidity and mortality in hypertension: the Captopril Prevention Project (CAPPP) randomised trial. Lancet 1999;353:611–616.
340. Curb JD, Pressel SL, Cutler JA, et al. Effect of diuretic-based antihypertensive treatment on cardiovascular disease risk in older diabetic patients with isolated systolic hypertension. Systolic Hypertension in the Elderly Program Cooperative Research Group. JAMA 1996;276:1886–1892.
341. UK Prospective Diabetes Study Group. Tight blood pressure control and risk of macrovascular and microvascular complications in type 2 diabetes: UKPDS 38. BMJ 1998;317:703–713.
342. Williams B, Poulter NR, Brown MJ, et al; BHS guidelines working party, for the British Hypertension Society. British Hypertension Society guidelines for hypertension management 2004 (BHS-IV): summary. BMJ 2004;328:634–640.
343. Adler AI, Stratton IM, Neil HA, et al. Association of systolic blood pressure with macrovascular and microvascular complications of type 2 diabetes (UKPDS 36): prospective observational study. BMJ 2000;321:412–419.
344. Culleton BF, Larson MG, Parfrey PS, et al. Proteinuria as a risk factor for cardiovascular disease and mortality in older people: a prospective study. Am J Med 2000;109:1–8.
345. K/DOQI clinical practice guidelines on hypertension and antihypertensive agents in chronic kidney disease. Am J Kidney Dis 2004;43:S1–S290.
346. Antithrombotic Trialists' Collaboration. Collaborative meta-analysis of randomised trials of antiplatelet therapy for prevention of death, myocardial infarction, and stroke in high risk patients. BMJ 2002;324:71–86.
347. Sanmuganathan PS, Ghahramani P, Jackson PR, et al. Aspirin for primary prevention of coronary heart disease: safety and absolute benefit related to coronary risk derived from meta-analysis of randomised trials. Heart 2001;85:265–271.
348. Patrono C, Bachmann F, Baigent C, et al. Expert consensus document on the use of antiplatelet agents: the task force on the use of antiplatelet agents in patients with atherosclerotic cardiovascular disease of the European Society of Cardiology. Eur Heart J 2004;25:166–181.
349. Saloheimo P, Juvela S, Hillbom M. Use of aspirin, epistaxis, and untreated hypertension as risk factors for primary intracerebral hemorrhage in middle-aged and elderly people. Stroke 2001;32:399–404.
350. CAPRIE Steering Committee. A randomised, blinded, trial of clopidogrel versus aspirin in patients at risk of ischaemic events (CAPRIE). Lancet 1996;348:1329–1339.
351. Yusuf S, Zhao F, Mehta SR, et al; Clopidogrel in Unstable Angina to Prevent Recurrent Events Trial Investigators. Effects of clopidogrel in addition to aspirin in patients with acute coronary syndromes without ST-segment elevation. N Engl J Med 2001;345:494–502.
352. Bhatt DL, Topol EJ, on behalf of the CHARISMA Executive Committee. Clopidogrel added to aspirin versus aspirin alone in secondary prevention and high-risk primary prevention: rationale and design of the clopidogrel for high atherothrombotic risk and ischemic stabilization, management and avoidance (CHARISMA) trial. Am Heart J 2004;148:263–268.
353. ESPS-2 Working Group. Second European Stroke Prevention Study. J Neurol 1992;239:299–301.
354. Jamieson DG, Parekh A, Ezekowitz MD. Review of antiplatelet therapy in secondary prevention of cerebrovascular events: a need for direct comparisons between antiplatelet agents. J Cardiovasc Pharmacol Ther 2005;10:153–161.
355. Stephenson BJ, Rowe BH, Haynes RB, et al. Is this patient taking the treatment as prescribed? JAMA 1993;269:2779–2781.
356. Bakris GL. The role of combination antihypertensive therapy and the progression of renal disease hypertension: looking toward the next millennium. Am J Hypertens 1998;11:158S–162S.
357. Yusuf S. Two decades of progress in preventing vascular disease. Lancet 2002;360:2–3.

147

Index

Notes: As the subject of this book is cardiovascular disease and risk management, all entries refer to these subjects unless stated otherwise. Page numbers in *italics* refer to figures. CS next to a page number indicates a case study. Abbreviations used in the index can be found on pages 129-132.

THE SILVER BOX

A COMEDY IN THREE ACTS

BY

JOHN GALSWORTHY

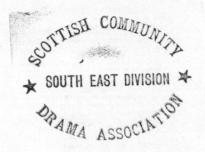

DUCKWORTH
HENRIETTA STREET, LONDON, W.C.

Published in	*1911*
Reprinted .	*1911*
,,	. *1912*
,,	. *1913*
,,	. *1913*
,,	. *1915*
,,	. *1917*
,,	. *1919*
,,	. *1920*
,,	. *1923*
,,	. *1923*
,,	. *1924*
,,	. *1925*
,,	. *1926*
,,	. *1929*

Made and Printed in Great Britain
by Turnbull & Spears, Edinburgh

PERSONS OF THE PLAY

JOHN BARTHWICK, M.P., *a wealthy Liberal*
MRS. BARTHWICK, *his wife*
JACK BARTHWICK, *their son*
ROPER, *their solicitor*
MRS. JONES, *their charwoman*
MARLOW, *their manservant*
WHEELER, *their maidservant*
JONES, *the stranger within their gates*
MRS. SEDDON, *a landlady*
SNOW, *a detective*
A POLICE MAGISTRATE
AN UNKNOWN LADY, *from beyond*
TWO LITTLE GIRLS, *homeless*
LIVENS, *their father*
A RELIEVING OFFICER
A MAGISTRATE'S CLERK
AN USHER
POLICEMEN, CLERKS, AND OTHERS

TIME: The present. The action of the first two Acts takes place on Easter Tuesday; the action of the third on Easter Wednesday week.

ACT I., SCENE I. *Rockingham Gate. John Barthwick's dining-room.*

   SCENE II. *The same.*

   SCENE III. *The same.*

ACT II., SCENE I. *The Jones' lodgings, Merthyr Street.*

   SCENE II. *John Barthwick's dining-room.*

ACT III. *A London police court.*

CAST OF THE ORIGINAL PRODUCTION AT THE ROYAL COURT THEATRE, LONDON, ON SEPTEMBER 25, 1906

JOHN BARTHWICK, M.P.	*Mr. James Hearn*
MRS. BARTHWICK	*Miss Frances Ivor*
JACK BARTHWICK	*Mr. A. E. Matthews*
ROPER	*Mr. A. Goodsall*
MRS. JONES	*Miss Irene Rooke*
MARLOW	*Mr. Frederick Lloyd*
WHEELER	*Miss Gertrude Henriques*
JONES	*Mr. Norman McKinnell*
MRS. SEDDON	*Mrs. Charles Maltby*
SNOW	*Mr. Trevor Lowe*
A POLICE MAGISTRATE	*Mr. Athol Forde*
AN UNKNOWN LADY	*Miss Sydney Fairbrother*
LIVENS	*Mr. Edmund Gurney*
RELIEVING OFFICER	*Mr. Edmund Gwenn*
MAGISTRATE'S CLERK	*Mr. Lewis Casson*
USHER	*Mr. Norman Page*

ACT I

SCENE I

The curtain rises on the BARTHWICKS' *dining-room, large,
modern, and well furnished ; the window curtains
drawn. Electric light is burning. On the large
round dining-table is set out a tray with whisky, a
syphon, and a silver cigarette-box. It is past midnight.*

*A fumbling is heard outside the door. It is opened sud-
denly ;* JACK BARTHWICK *seems to fall into the
room. He stands holding by the door knob, staring
before him, with a beatific smile. He is in evening
dress and opera hat, and carries in his hand a sky-
blue velvet lady's reticule. His boyish face is freshly
coloured and clean-shaven. An overcoat is hanging
on his arm.*

JACK. Hello ! I've got home all ri—— [*Defiantly.*]
Who says I sh'd never've opened th' door without
'sistance. [*He staggers in, fumbling with the reticule.
A lady's handkerchief and purse of crimson silk fall out.*]
Serve her joll' well right—everything droppin' out.
Th' cat. I've scored her off—I've got her bag. [*He
swings the reticule.*] Serves her joll' well right. [*He

5

takes a cigarette out of the silver box and puts it in his mouth.] Never gave tha' fellow anything! [*He hunts through all his pockets and pulls a shilling out; it drops and rolls away. He looks for it.*] Beastly shilling! [*He looks again.*] Base ingratitude! Absolutely nothing. [*He laughs.*] Mus' tell him I've got absolutely nothing.

> [*He lurches through the door and down a corridor, and presently returns, followed by* JONES, *who is advanced in liquor.* JONES, *about thirty years of age, has hollow cheeks, black circles round his eyes, and rusty clothes. He looks as though he might be unemployed, and enters in a hang-dog manner.*]

JACK. Sh! sh! sh! Don't you make a noise, whatever you do. Shu' the door, an' have a drink. [*Very solemnly.*] You helped me to open the door —I've got nothin' for you. This is my house. My father's name's Barthwick; he's Member of Parliament—Liberal Member of Parliament: I've told you that before. Have a drink! [*He pours out whisky and drinks it up.*] I'm not drunk—— [*Subsiding on a sofa.*] Tha's all right. Wha's your name? My name's Barthwick, so's my father's; *I'm* a Liberal too—wha're you?

JONES. [*In a thick, sardonic voice.*] I'm a bloomin' Conservative. My name's Jones! My wife works 'ere; she's the char; she works 'ere.

JACK. Jones? [*He laughs.*] There's 'nother Jones at college with me. I'm not a Socialist myself; I'm

a Liberal—there's ve-lill difference, because of the
principles of the Lib—Liberal Party. We're all
equal before the law—tha's rot, tha's silly. [*Laughs.*]
Wha' was I about to say? Give me some whisky.

> [JONES *gives him the whisky he desires, together
> with a squirt of syphon.*]

Wha' I was goin' tell you was—I've had a row with
her. [*He waves the reticule.*]   Have a drink, Jones—
sh'd never have got in without you—tha's why I'm
giving you a drink. Don' care who knows I've scored
her off. Th' cat! [*He throws his feet up on the sofa.*]
Don' you make a noise, whatever you do. You pour
out a drink—you make yourself good long, long drink
—you take cigarette—you take anything you like.
Sh'd never have got in without you. [*Closing his
eyes.*]   You're a Tory—you're a Tory Socialist. I'm
Liberal myself—have a drink—I'm an excel'nt chap.

> [*His head drops back. He, smiling, falls asleep,
> and* JONES *stands looking at him; then,
> snatching up* JACK's *glass, he drinks it off.
> He picks the reticule from off* JACK's *shirt-
> front, holds it to the light, and smells at it.*]

JONES. Been on the tiles and brought 'ome some
of yer cat's fur. [*He stuffs it into* JACK's *breast pocket.*]
JACK. [*Murmuring.*] I've scored you off! You cat!

> [JONES *looks around him furtively; he pours
> out whisky and drinks it. From the silver
> box he takes a cigarette, puffs at it, and drinks
> more whisky. There is no sobriety left in
> him.*]

JONES. Fat lot o' things they've got 'ere ! [*He sees the crimson purse lying on the floor.*] More cats' fur. Puss, puss ! [*He fingers it, drops it on the tray, and looks at* JACK.] Calf ! Fat calf ! [*He sees his own presentment in a mirror. Lifting his hands, with fingers spread, he stares at it ; then looks again at* JACK, *clenching his fist as if to batter in his sleeping, smiling face. Suddenly he tilts the rest of the whisky into the glass and drinks it. With cunning glee he takes the silver box and purse and pockets them.*] I'll score *you* off too, that's wot I'll do !

> [*He gives a little snarling laugh and lurches to the door. His shoulder rubs against the switch ; the light goes out. There is a sound as of a closing outer door.*

The curtain falls.

The curtain rises again at once.

SCENE II

In the BARTHWICKS' *dining-room.* JACK *is still asleep; the morning light is coming through the curtains. The time is half-past eight.* WHEELER, *brisk person, enters with a dust-pan, and* MRS. JONES *more slowly with a scuttle.*

WHEELER. [*Drawing the curtains.*] That precious husband of yours was round for you after you'd gone yesterday, Mrs. Jones. Wanted your money for drink, I suppose. He hangs about the corner here half the time.   I saw him outside the "Goat and Bells" when I went to the post last night.   If I were you I wouldn't live with him.   I wouldn't live with a man that raised his hand to me.   I wouldn't put up with it.   Why don't you take the children and leave him? If you put up with 'im it'll only make him worse.   I never can see why, because a man's married you, he should knock you about.

MRS. JONES. [*Slim, dark-eyed, and dark-haired; oval-faced, and with a smooth, soft, even voice ; her manner patient, her way of talking quite impersonal; she wears a blue linen dress, and boots with holes.*] It was nearly two last night before he come home, and he wasn't himself.   He made me get up, and he knocked me about; he didn't seem to know *what* he was saying or doing.   Of course I *would* leave him, but I'm really afraid of what he'd do to me.   He's such a violent man when he's not himself.

WHEELER. Why don't you get him locked up? You'll never have any peace until you get him locked up.   If I were you I'd go to the police court to-morrow.   That's what I would do.

MRS. JONES. Of course I ought to go, because he does treat me so badly when he's not himself.   But you see, Bettina, he has a very hard time—he's been out of work two months, and it preys upon his mind. When he's in work he behaves himself much better. It's when he's out of work that he's so violent.

WHEELER. Well, if you won't take any steps you'll never get rid of him.

MRS. JONES. Of course it's very wearing to me; I don't get my sleep at nights. And it's not as if I were getting help from him, because I have to do for the children and all of us. And he throws such dreadful things up at me, talks of my having men to follow me about. Such a thing never happens; no man ever speaks to me. And of course it's just the other way. It's what he does that's wrong and makes me so unhappy. And then he's always threatenin' to cut my throat if I leave him. It's all the drink, and things preying on his mind; he's not a bad man really. Sometimes he'll speak quite kind to me, but I've stood so much from him, I don't feel it in me to speak kind back, but just keep myself to myself. And he's all right with the children too, except when he's not himself.

WHEELER. You mean when he's drunk, the beauty.

MRS. JONES. Yes. [*Without change of voice.*] There's the young gentleman asleep on the sofa.

> [*They both look silently at Jack.*

MRS. JONES. [*At last, in her soft voice.*] He doesn't look quite himself.

WHEELER. He's a young limp. that's what he is. It's my belief he was tipsy last night, like your husband. It's another kind of bein' out of work that sets *him* to drink. I'll go and tell Marlow. This is his job.   [*She goes.*

> [*Mrs. Jones, upon her knees, begins a gentle sweeping.*

JACK. [*Waking.*] Who's there ? What is it ?

MRS. JONES. It's me, sir, Mrs. Jones.

JACK. [*Sitting up and looking round.*] Where is it—what—what time is it?

MRS. JONES. It's getting on for nine o'clock, sir.

JACK. For nine! Why—what! [*Rising, and loosening his tongue; putting hand to his head, and staring hard at Mrs. Jones.*] Look here, you, Mrs.—Mrs. Jones—don't you say you caught me asleep here.

MRS. JONES. No, sir, of course I won't, sir.

JACK. It's quite an accident; I don't know how it happened. I must have forgotten to go to bed. It's a queer thing. I've got a most beastly headache. Mind you don't say anything, Mrs. Jones.

> [*Goes out and passes MARLOW in the doorway. MARLOW is young and quiet; he is clean-shaven, and his hair is brushed high from his forehead in a coxcomb. Incidentally a butler, he is first a man. He looks at MRS. JONES, and smiles a private smile.*

MARLOW. Not the first time, and won't be the last. Looked a bit dicky, eh, Mrs. Jones?

MRS. JONES. He didn't look quite himself. Of course I didn't take notice.

MARLOW. You're used to them. How's your old man?

MRS. JONES. [*Softly as throughout.*] Well, he was very bad last night; he didn't seem to know what he was about. He was very late, and he was most abusive. But now, of course, he's asleep.

MARLOW. That's his way of finding a job, eh?

MRS. JONES. As a rule, Mr. Marlow, he goes out

early every morning looking for work, and sometimes he comes in fit to drop—and of course I can't say he doesn't try to get it, because he does. Trade's very bad. [*She stands quite still, her pan and brush before her, at the beginning and the end of long vistas of experience, traversing them with her impersonal eye.*] But he's not a good husband to me—last night he hit me, and he was so dreadfully abusive.

MARLOW. Bank 'oliday, eh! He's too fond of the "Goat and Bells," that's what's the matter with him. I see him at the corner late every night. He hangs about.

MRS. JONES. He gets to feeling very low walking about all day after work, and being refused so often, and then when he gets a drop in him it goes to his head. But he shouldn't treat his wife as he treats me. Sometimes I've had to go and walk about at night, when he wouldn't let me stay in the room; but he's sorry for it afterwards. And he hangs about after me, he waits for me in the street; and I don't think he ought to, because I've always been a good wife to him. And I tell him Mrs. Barthwick wouldn't like him coming about the place. But that only makes him angry, and he says dreadful things about the gentry. Of course it was through me that he first lost his place, through his not treating me right; and that's made him bitter against the gentry. He had a very good place as groom in the country; but it made such a stir, because of course he didn't treat me right.

MARLOW. Got the sack?

MRS. JONES. Yes; his employer said he couldn't keep him, because there was a great deal of talk; and he said it was such a bad example. But it's very important for me to keep my work here; I have the three children, and I don't want him to come about after me in the streets, and make a disturbance as he sometimes does.

MARLOW. [*Holding up the empty decanter.*] Not a drain! Next time he hits you get a witness and go down to the court——

MRS. JONES. Yes, I think I've made up my mind. I think I ought to.

MARLOW. That's right. Where's the ciga——?

[*He searches for the silver box; he looks at MRS. JONES, who is sweeping on her hands and knees; he checks himself and stands reflecting. From the tray he picks two half-smoked cigarettes, and reads the name of them.*

Nestor—where the deuce——?

[*With a meditative air he looks again at MRS. JONES, and, taking up JACK's overcoat, he searches in the pockets. WHEELER, with a tray of breakfast things, comes in.*

MARLOW. [*Aside to WHEELER.*] Have you seen the cigarette-box?

WHEELER. No.

MARLOW. Well, it's gone. I put it on the tray last night. And he's been smoking. [*Showing her the ends of cigarette.*] It's not in these pockets. He can't have taken it upstairs this morning! Have a good look in his room when he comes down. Who's been in here?

WHEELER. Only me and Mrs. Jones.

MRS. JONES. I've finished here; shall I do the drawing-room now?

WHEELER. [*Looking at her doubtfully.*] Have you seen—— Better do the boudwower first.

> [MRS. JONES *goes out with pan and brush.*
> MARLOW *and* WHEELER *look each other in the face.*

MARLOW. It'll turn up.

WHEELER. [*Hesitating.*] You don't think *she*—— [*Nodding at the door.*]

MARLOW. [*Stoutly.*] I don't—I never believes anything of anybody.

WHEELER. But the master'll have to be told.

MARLOW. You wait a bit, and see if it don't turn up. Suspicion's no business of ours. I set my mind against it.

The curtain falls.

The curtain rises again at once

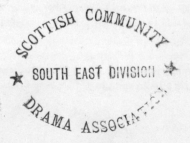

SCENE III

BARTHWICK *and* MRS. BARTHWICK *are seated at the breakfast table. He is a man between fifty and sixty;
quietly important, with a bald forehead, and pince-
nez, and the " Times" in his hand. She is a lady of
nearly fifty, well dressed, with greyish hair, good features, and a decided manner. They face each other.*

BARTHWICK. [*From behind his paper.*] The Labour
man has got in at the by-election for Barnside, my
dear.

MRS. BARTHWICK. Another Labour ?   I can't think
what on earth the country is about.

BARTHWICK. I predicted it.   It's not a matter of
vast importance.

MRS. BARTHWICK. Not ?   How can you take it so
calmly, John ?   To me it's simply outrageous.   And
there you sit, you Liberals, and pretend to encourage
these people !

BARTHWICK. [*Frowning.*] The representation of all
parties is necessary for any proper reform, for any
proper social policy.

MRS. BARTHWICK. I've no patience with your talk of
reform—all that nonsense about social policy.   We
know perfectly well what it is they want ; they want
things for themselves.   Those Socialists and Labour
men are an absolutely selfish set of people.   They
have no sense of patriotism, like the upper classes,
they simply want what we've got.

B

BARTHWICK. Want what we've got! [*He stares into space.*] My dear, what are you talking about? [*With a contortion.*] I'm no alarmist.

MRS. BARTHWICK. Cream? Quite uneducated men! Wait until they begin to tax our investments. I'm convinced that when they once get a chance they will tax everything—they've no feeling for the country. You Liberals and Conservatives, you're all alike ; you don't see an inch before your noses. You've no imagination, not a scrap of imagination between you. You ought to join hands and nip it in the bud.

BARTHWICK. You're talking nonsense! How is it possible for Liberals and Conservatives to join hands, as you call it? That shows how absurd it is for women—— Why, the very essence of a Liberal is to trust in the people!

MRS. BARTHWICK. Now, John, eat your breakfast. As if there were any real difference between you and the Conservatives. All the upper classes have the same interests to protect, and the same principles. [*Calmly.*] Oh! you're sitting upon a volcano, John.

BARTHWICK. What!

MRS. BARTHWICK. I read a letter in the paper yesterday. I forget the man's name, but it made the whole thing perfectly clear. You don't look things in the face.

BARTHWICK. Indeed! [*Heavily.*] I am a Liberal! Drop the subject, please!

MRS. BARTHWICK. Toast? I quite agree with what this man says : Education is simply ruining the lower

classes. It unsettles them, and that's the worst thing
for us all. I see an enormous difference in the manner
of servants.

BARTHWICK. [*With suspicious emphasis.*] I welcome
any change that will lead to something better. [*He
opens a letter.*] H'm! This is that affair of Master
Jack's again. " High Street, Oxford. Sir, We have
received Mr. John Barthwick, Senior's, draft for forty
pounds." Oh! the letter's to him! " We now en-
close the cheque you cashed with us, which, as we
stated in our previous letter, was not met on pre-
sentation at your bank. We are, Sir, yours obediently,
Moss and Sons, Tailors." H'm! [*Staring at the
cheque.*] A pretty business altogether! The boy
might have been prosecuted.

MRS. BARTHWICK. Come, John, you know Jack
didn't mean anything; he only thought he was over-
drawing. I still think his bank ought to have cashed
that cheque. They must know your position.

BARTHWICK. [*Replacing in the envelope the letter and
the cheque.*] Much good that would have done him
in a court of law. [*He stops as* JACK *comes in, fasten-
ing his waistcoat and staunching a razor cut upon his
chin.*]

JACK. [*Sitting down between them, and speaking with
an artificial joviality.*] Sorry I'm late. [*He looks
lugubriously at the dishes.*] Tea, please, mother. Any
letters for me? [BARTHWICK *hands the letter to him.*]
But look here, I say, this has been opened! I do
wish you wouldn't——

BARTHWICK. [*Touching the envelope.*] I suppose I'm entitled to this name.

JACK. [*Sulkily.*] Well, I can't help having your name, father! [*He reads the letter, and mutters.*] Brutes

BARTHWICK. [*Eyeing him.*] You don't deserve to be so well out of that.

JACK. Haven't you ragged me enough, dad?

MRS. BARTHWICK. Yes, John, let Jack have his breakfast.

BARTHWICK. If you hadn't had me to come to, where would you have been? It's the merest accident—suppose you had been the son of a poor man or a clerk. Obtaining money with a cheque you knew your bank could not meet. It might have ruined you for life. I can't see what's to become of you if these are your principles. I never did anything of the sort myself.

JACK. I expect you always had lots of money. If you've got plenty of money, of course——

BARTHWICK. On the contrary, I had not your advantages. My father kept me very short of money.

JACK. How much had you, dad?

BARTHWICK. It's not material. The question is, do you feel the gravity of what you did?

JACK. I don't know about the gravity. Of course, I'm very sorry if you think it was wrong. Haven't I said so! I should never have done it at all if I hadn't been so jolly hard up.

BARTHWICK. How much of that forty pounds have you got left, Jack?

JACK. [*Hesitating.*] I don't know—not much.

BARTHWICK. How much?

JACK. [*Desperately.*] I haven't got any.

BARTHWICK. What?

JACK. I know I've got the most beastly headache.

[*He leans his head on his hand.*

MRS. BARTHWICK. Headache? My dear boy! Can't you eat any breakfast?

JACK. [*Drawing in his breath.*] Too jolly bad!

MRS. BARTHWICK. I'm so sorry. Come with me, dear; I'll give you something that will take it away at once.

[*They leave the room; and* BARTHWICK, *tearing up the letter, goes to the fireplace and puts the pieces in the fire. While he is doing this* MARLOW *comes in, and, looking round him, is about quietly to withdraw.*

BARTHWICK. What's that? What d'you want?

MARLOW. I was looking for Mr. John, sir.

BARTHWICK. What d'you want Mr. John for?

MARLOW. [*With hesitation.*] I thought I should find him here, sir.

BARTHWICK. [*Suspiciously.*] Yes, but what do you want him for?

MARLOW. [*Offhandedly.*] There's a lady called— asked to speak to him for a minute, sir.

BARTHWICK. A lady, at this time in the morning. What sort of a lady?

MARLOW. [*Without expression in his voice.*] I can't tell, sir; no particular sort. She might be after charity. She might be a Sister of Mercy, I should think, sir.

BARTHWICK. Is she dressed like one ?

MARLOW. No, sir, she's in plain clothes, sir.

BARTHWICK. Didn't she say what she wanted ?

MARLOW. No, sir.

BARTHWICK. Where did you leave her ?

MARLOW. In the hall, sir.

BARTHWICK. In the hall ? How do you know she's not a thief—not got designs on the house?

MARLOW. No, sir, I don't fancy so, sir.

BARTHWICK. Well, show her in here ; I'll see her myself.

> [MARLOW *goes out with a private gesture of dis-*
> *may. He soon returns, ushering in a young*
> *pale lady with dark eyes and pretty figure, in*
> *a modish, black, but rather shabby dress, a*
> *black and white trimmed hat with a bunch of*
> *Parma violets wrongly placed, and fuzzy-*
> *spotted veil. At the sight of* MR. BARTHWICK
> *she exhibits every sign of nervousness.* MAR-
> LOW *goes out.*

UNKNOWN LADY. Oh ! but—I beg pardon—there's some mistake— I—— [*She turns to fly.*]

BARTHWICK. Whom did you want to see, madam ?

UNKNOWN. [*Stopping and looking back.*] It was Mr. *John* Barthwick I wanted to see.

BARTHWICK. I am John Barthwick, madam. What can I have the pleasure of doing for you ?

UNKNOWN. Oh ! I—I don't—— [*She drops her*

eyes.   BARTHWICK *scrutinises her, and purses his lips.*]

BARTHWICK. It was my son, perhaps, you wished to see ?

UNKNOWN. [*Quickly.*] Yes, of course, it's your son.

BARTHWICK. May I ask whom I have the pleasure of speaking to ?

UNKNOWN. [*Appeal and hardiness upon her face.*] My name is—oh ! it doesn't matter—I don't want to make any fuss. I just want to see your son for a minute. [*Boldly.*] In fact, I *must* see him.

BARTHWICK. [*Controlling his uneasiness.*] My son is not very well. If necessary, no doubt I could attend to the matter ; be so kind as to let me know——

UNKNOWN. Oh ! but I *must* see him—I've come on purpose——[*She bursts out nervously.*] I don't want to make any fuss, but the fact is, last— last night your son took away—he took away my—— [*She stops.*]

BARTHWICK. [*Severely.*] Yes, madam, what ?

UNKNOWN. He took away my—my reticule.

BARTHWICK. Your reti——?

UNKNOWN. I don't care about the reticule ; it's not *that* I want—I'm sure I don't want to make any fuss—[*her face is quivering*]—but—but—all my money was in it !

BARTHWICK. In what—in what ?

UNKNOWN. In my purse, in the reticule. It was a crimson silk purse. Really, I wouldn't have come— I don't want to make any fuss. But I must get my money back—mustn't I ?

BARTHWICK. Do you tell me that my son——?

UNKNOWN. Oh! well you see, he wasn't quite—I mean he was——   [*She smiles mesmerically.*

BARTHWICK. I beg your pardon.

UNKNOWN. [*Stamping her foot.*] Oh! don't you see—tipsy! We had a quarrel.

BARTHWICK. [*Scandalised.*] How? Where?

UNKNOWN. [*Defiantly.*] At my place. We'd had supper at the——and your son——

BARTHWICK. [*Pressing the bell.*] May I ask how you knew this house? Did he give you his name and address?

UNKNOWN. [*Glancing sidelong.*] I got it out of his overcoat.

BARTHWICK. [*Sardonically.*] Oh! you got it out of his overcoat. And may I ask if my son will know you by daylight?

UNKNOWN. Know me? I should jolly—I mean, of course he will!   [MARLOW *comes in.*

BARTHWICK. Ask Mr. John to come down.

[MARLOW *goes out, and* BARTHWICK *walks uneasily about.*

And how long have you enjoyed his acquaintanceship?

UNKNOWN. Only since—only since Good Friday.

BARTHWICK. I am at a loss—I repeat I am at a loss——

[*He glances at this unknown lady, who stands with eyes cast down, twisting her hands. And suddenly Jack appears. He stops on seeing*

who is here, and the unknown lady hys-
terically giggles. There is a silence.

BARTHWICK. [*Portentously.*] This young—er—lady
says that last night—I think you said last night,
madam—you took away——

UNKNOWN. [*Impulsively.*] My reticule, and all my
money was in a crimson silk purse.

JACK. Reticule. [*Looking round for any chance to
get away.*] I don't know anything about it.

BARTHWICK. [*Sharply.*] Come, do you deny seeing
this young lady last night?

JACK. Deny? No, of course. [*Whispering.*] Why
did you give me away like this? What on earth did
you come here for?

UNKNOWN. [*Tearfully.*] I'm sure I didn't want to—
it's not likely, is it? You snatched it out of my hand—
you know you did—and the purse had all my money in
it. I didn't follow you last night because I didn't want
to make a fuss and it was so late, and you were so——

BARTHWICK. Come, sir, don't turn your back on
me—explain!

JACK. [*Desperately.*] I don't remember anything
about it. [*In a low voice to his friend.*] Why on earth
couldn't you have written?

UNKNOWN. [*Sullenly.*] I want it now; I must have
it—I've got to pay my rent to-day. [*She looks at
BARTHWICK.*] They're only too glad to jump on people
who are not—not *well off*.

JACK. I don't remember anything about it, really.
I don't remember anything about last night at all.

[*He puts his hand up to his head.*] It's all—cloudy, and I've got such a beastly headache.

UNKNOWN. But you *took* it; you know you did. You said you'd score me off.

JACK. Well, then, it must be here. I remember now—I remember something. Why did I take the beastly thing?

BARTHWICK. Yes, why did you take the beastly——
                    [*He turns abruptly to the window.*

UNKNOWN. [*With her mesmeric smile.*] You weren't quite——were you?

JACK. [*Smiling pallidly.*] I'm *awfully* sorry. If there's anything I can do——

BARTHWICK. Do? You can restore this property, I suppose.

JACK. I'll go and have a look, but I really don't think I've got it.

> [*He goes out hurriedly. And* BARTHWICK, *placing a chair, motions to the visitor to sit; then, with pursed lips, he stands and eyes her fixedly. She sits, and steals a look at him; then turns away, and, drawing up her veil, stealthily wipes her eyes. And* JACK *comes back.*

JACK. [*Ruefully holding out the empty reticule.*] Is that the thing? I've looked all over—I can't find the purse anywhere. Are you sure it was there?

UNKNOWN. [*Tearfully.*] Sure? Of course I'm sure. A crimson silk purse. It was all the money I had.

JACK. I really am awfully sorry—my head's so jolly bad. I've asked the butler, but he hasn't seen it.

UNKNOWN. I *must* have my money——

JACK. Oh! Of course—that'll be all right; I'll see that that's all right. How much?

UNKNOWN. [*Sullenly.*] Seven pounds—twelve—it's all I've got in the world.

JACK. That'll be all right; I'll—send you a—cheque.

UNKNOWN. [*Eagerly.*] No; now, please. Give me what was in my purse; I've got to pay my rent this morning. They won't give me another day; I'm a fortnight behind already.

JACK. [*Blankly.*] I'm awfully sorry; I really haven't a penny in my pocket.

[*He glances stealthily at* BARTHWICK.

UNKNOWN. [*Excitedly.*] Come, I say you must—it's my money, and you took it. I'm not going away without it. They'll turn me out of my place.

JACK. [*Clasping his head.*] But I can't give you what I haven't got. Don't I tell you I haven't a beastly penny?

UNKNOWN. [*Tearing at her handkerchief.*] Oh! do give it me! [*She puts her hands together in appeal; then, with sudden fierceness.*] If you don't I'll summons you. It's stealing, that's what it is!

BARTHWICK. [*Uneasily.*] One moment, please. As a matter of—er—principle, I shall settle this claim. [*He produces money.*] Here is eight pounds; the extra will cover the value of the purse and your cab fares. I need make no comment—no thanks are necessary.

> [*Touching the bell, he holds the door ajar in silence. The Unknown lady stores the money in her reticule, she looks from* JACK *to* BARTHWICK, *and her face is quivering faintly with a smile. She hides it with her hand, and steals away. Behind her* BARTHWICK *shuts the door.*

BARTHWICK. [*With solemnity.*] H'm! This is a nice thing to happen!

JACK. [*Impersonally.*] What awful luck!

BARTHWICK. So this is the way that forty pounds has gone! One thing after another! Once more I should like to know where you'd have been if it hadn't been for me! You don't seem to have any principles. You —you're one of those who are a nuisance to society; you—you're dangerous! What your mother would say I don't know. Your conduct, as far as I can see, is absolutely unjustifiable. It's—it's criminal. Why, a poor man who behaved as you've done . . .d'you think he'd have any mercy shown him? What you want is a good lesson. You and your sort are—[*he speaks with feeling*]—a nuisance to the community. Don't ask me to help you next time. You're not fit to be helped.

JACK. [*Turning upon his sire, with unexpected fierceness.*] All right, I won't then, and see how you like it. You wouldn't have helped me this time, I know, if you hadn't been scared the thing would get into the papers. Where are the cigarettes?

BARTHWICK. [*Regarding him uneasily.*]   Well—I'll say no more about it.   [*He rings the bell.*]   I'll pass it over for this once, but——   [MARLOW *comes in.* You can clear away.

                [*He hides his face behind the " Times."*

JACK. [*Brightening.*] I say, Marlow, where are the cigarettes ?

MARLOW. I put the box out with the whisky last night, sir, but this morning I can't find it anywhere.

JACK. Did you look in my room ?

MARLOW. Yes, sir ; l've looked all over the house. I found two Nestor ends in the tray this morning, so you must have been smokin' last night, sir. [*Hesitating.*] I'm really afraid some one's purloined the box.

JACK. [*Uneasily.*] Stolen it !

BARTHWICK. What's that ?   The cigarette-box ! Is anything else missing ?

MARLOW. No, sir ; I've been through the plate.

BARTHWICK. Was the house all right this morning ? None of the windows open ?

MARLOW. No, sir.   [*Quietly to* JACK.]   You left your latchkey in the door last night, sir.

            [*He hands it back, unseen by* BARTHWICK.
JACK. Tst !

BARTHWICK. Who's been in the room this morning ?

MARLOW. Me and Wheeler, and Mrs. Jones is all, sir, as far as I know.

BARTHWICK. Have you asked Mrs. Barthwick ? [*To* JACK.] Go and ask your mother if she's had it ;

ask her to look and see if she's missed anything
else.   [JACK *goes upon this mission.*
Nothing is more disquieting than losing things like this.

MARLOW. No, sir.

BARTHWICK. Have you any suspicions?

MARLOW. No, sir.

BARTHWICK. This Mrs. Jones—how long has she
been working here?

MARLOW. Only this last month, sir.

BARTHWICK. What sort of person?

MARLOW. I don't know much about her, sir;
seems a very quiet, respectable woman.

BARTHWICK. Who did the room this morning?

MARLOW. Wheeler and Mrs. Jones, sir.

BARTHWICK. [*With his forefinger upraised.*] Now, was
this Mrs. Jones in the room alone at any time?

MARLOW. [*Expressionless.*] Yes, sir.

BARTHWICK. How do you know that?

MARLOW. [*Reluctantly.*] I found her here, sir.

BARTHWICK. And has Wheeler been in the room
alone?

MARLOW. No, sir, she's not, sir. I should say, sir,
that Mrs. Jones seems a very honest——

BARTHWICK. [*Holding up his hand.*] I want to know
this: Has this Mrs. Jones been here the whole
morning?

MARLOW. Yes, sir—no, sir—she stepped over to the
greengrocer's for cook.

BARTHWICK. H'm! Is she in the house now?

MARLOW. Yes, sir.

BARTHWICK. Very good. I shall make a point of clearing this up. On principle I shall make a point of fixing the responsibility ; it goes to the foundations of security. In all your interests——

MARLOW. Yes, sir.

BARTHWICK. What sort of circumstances is this Mrs. Jones in ? Is her husband in work ?

MARLOW. I believe not, sir.

BARTHWICK. Very well. Say nothing about it to any one. Tell Wheeler not to speak of it, and ask Mrs. Jones to step up here.

MARLOW. Very good, sir.

> [MARLOW *goes out, his face concerned ; and* BARTHWICK *stays, his face judicial and a little pleased, as befits a man conducting an inquiry.* MRS. BARTHWICK *and her son come in.*

BARTHWICK. Well, my dear, you've not seen it, I suppose ?

MRS. BARTHWICK. No. But what an extraordinary thing, John ! Marlow, of course, is out of the question. I'm certain none of the maids——As for cook !

BARTHWICK. Oh, cook !

MRS. BARTHWICK. Of course ! It's perfectly detestable to me to suspect anybody.

BARTHWICK. It is not a question of one's feelings. It's a question of justice. On principle——

MRS. BARTHWICK. I shouldn't be a bit surprised if the charwoman knew something about it. It was Laura who recommended her.

BARTHWICK. [*Judicially.*] I am going to have Mrs. Jones up. Leave it to me; and—er—remember that nobody is guilty until they're proved so. I shall be careful. I have no intention of frightening her; I shall give her every chance. I hear she's in poor circumstances. If we are not able to do much for them we are bound to have the greatest sympathy with the poor.   [MRS. JONES *comes in.*
[*Pleasantly.*] Oh! good morning, Mrs. Jones.

MRS. JONES. [*Soft, and even, unemphatic.*] Good morning, sir! Good morning, ma'am!

BARTHWICK. About your husband—he's not in work, I hear?

MRS. JONES. No, sir; of course he's not in work just now.

BARTHWICK. Then I suppose he's earning nothing.

MRS. JONES. No, sir, he's not earning anything just now, sir.

BARTHWICK. And how many children have you?

MRS. JONES. Three children; but of course they don't eat very much, sir.   [*A little silence.*

BARTHWICK. And how old is the eldest?

MRS. JONES. Nine years old, sir.

BARTHWICK. Do they go to school?

MRS. JONES. Yes, sir, they all three go to school every day.

BARTHWICK. [*Severely.*] And what about their food when you're out at work.

MRS. JONES. Well, sir, I have to give them their dinner to take with them. Of course I'm not always able to give them anything; sometimes I have to send them without; but my husband is very good about the children when he's in work. But when he's not in work of course he's a very difficult man.

BARTHWICK. He drinks, I suppose?

MRS. JONES. Yes, sir. Of course I can't say he doesn't drink, because he does.

BARTHWICK. And I suppose he takes all your money?

MRS. JONES. No, sir, he's very good about my money, except when he's not himself, and then, of course, he treats me very badly.

BARTHWICK. Now what is he—your husband?

MRS. JONES. By profession, sir, of course he's a groom.

BARTHWICK. A groom! How came he to lose his place?

MRS. JONES. He lost his place a long time ago, sir, and he's never had a very long job since; and now, of course, the motor-cars are against him.

BARTHWICK. When were you married to him, Mrs. Jones?

MRS. JONES. Eight years ago, sir—that was in——

MRS. BARTHWICK. [Sharply.] Eight? You said the eldest child was nine.

MRS. JONES. Yes, ma'am; of course that was why he lost his place. He didn't treat me rightly, and of course his employer said he couldn't keep him because of the example.

BARTHWICK.   You mean he—ahem——

C

MRS. JONES. Yes, sir; and of course after he lost his place he married me.

MRS. BARTHWICK. You actually mean to say you— you were——

BARTHWICK. My dear——

MRS. BARTHWICK. [*Indignantly.*] How disgraceful!

BARTHWICK. [*Hurriedly.*] And where are you living now, Mrs. Jones?

MRS. JONES. We've not got a home, sir. Of course we've been obliged to put away most of our things.

BARTHWICK. Put your things away! You mean to —to—er—to pawn them?

MRS. JONES. Yes, sir, to put them away. We're living in Merthyr Street—that is close by here, sir— at No. 34. We just have the one room.

BARTHWICK. And what do you pay a week?

MRS. JONES. We pay six shillings a week, sir, for a furnished room.

BARTHWICK. And I suppose you're behind in the rent?

MRS. JONES. Yes, sir, we're a little behind in the rent.

BARTHWICK. But *you're* in good work, aren't you?

MRS. JONES. Well, sir, I have a day in Stamford Place Thursdays. And Mondays and Wednesdays and Fridays I come here. But to-day, of course, is a half-day, because of yesterday's Bank Holiday.

BARTHWICK. I see; four days a week, and you get half a crown a day, is that it?

MRS. JONES. Yes, sir, and my dinner; but sometimes it's only half a day, and that's eighteenpence.

BARTHWICK. And when your husband earns anything he spends it in drink, I suppose?

MRS. JONES. Sometimes he does, sir, and sometimes he gives it to me for the children. Of course he would work if he could get it, sir, but it seems there are a great many people out of work.

BARTHWICK. Ah! Yes. We—er—won't go into that. [*Sympathetically.*] And how about your work here? Do you find it hard?

MRS. JONES. Oh! no, sir, not very hard, sir; except of course, when I don't get my sleep at night.

BARTHWICK. Ah! And you help do all the rooms? And sometimes, I suppose, you go out for cook?

MRS. JONES. Yes, sir.

BARTHWICK. And you've been out this morning?

MRS. JONES. Yes, sir, of course I had to go to the greengrocer's.

BARTHWICK. Exactly. So your husband earns nothing? And he's a bad character.

MRS. JONES. No, sir, I don't say that, sir. I think there's a great deal of good in him; though he does treat me very bad sometimes. And of course I don't like to leave him, but I think I ought to, because really I hardly know how to stay with him. He often raises his hand to me. Not long ago he gave me a blow here [*touches her breast*] and I can feel it now. So I think I ought to leave him, don't *you*, sir?

BARTHWICK. Ah! I can't help you there. It's a very serious thing to leave your husband. Very serious thing.

MRS. JONES. Yes, sir, of course I'm afraid of what he might do to me if I were to leave him; he can be so very violent.

BARTHWICK. H'm! Well, that I can't pretend to say anything about. It's the bad principle I'm speaking of—

MRS. JONES. Yes, sir; I know nobody can help me. I know I must decide for myself, and of course I know that he has a very hard life. And he's fond of the children, and it's very hard for him to see them going without food.

BARTHWICK. [*Hastily.*] Well—er—thank you, I just wanted to hear about you. I don't think I need detain you any longer, Mrs.—Jones.

MRS. JONES. No, sir, thank you, sir.

BARTHWICK. Good morning, then.

MRS. JONES. Good morning, sir; good morning, ma'am.

BARTHWICK. [*Exchanging glances with his wife.*] By the way, Mrs. Jones—I think it is only fair to tell you, a silver cigarette box—er—is missing.

MRS. JONES. [*Looking from one face to the other.*] I am very sorry, sir.

BARTHWICK. Yes; you have not seen it, I suppose?

MRS JONES. [*Realising that suspicion is upon her;*

with an uneasy movement.]   Where was it, sir; if you please, sir?

BARTHWICK. [*Evasively.*]   Where did Marlow say? Er—in this room, yes, in *this* room.

MRS. JONES. No, sir, I haven't seen it—of course if I'd seen it I should have noticed it.

BARTHWICK. [*Giving her a rapid glance.*]   You—you are sure of that?

MRS. JONES. [*Impassively.*]   Yes, sir. [*With a slow nodding of her head.*]   I have not seen it, and of course I *don't* know where it is.

> [*She turns and goes quietly out.*

BARTHWICK. H'm!

[*The three* BARTHWICKS *avoid each other's glances.*]

The curtain falls.

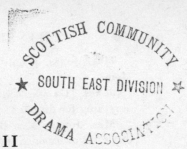

ACT II

SCENE I

The JONES' *lodgings, Merthyr Street, at half-past two*
o'clock.

The bare room, with tattered oilcloth and damp, dis-
tempered walls, has an air of tidy wretchedness.
On the bed lies JONES, *half-dressed; his coat is*
thrown across his feet, and muddy boots are lying
on the floor close by. He is asleep. The door is
opened and MRS. JONES *comes in, dressed in a*
pinched black jacket and old black sailor hat; she
carries a parcel wrapped up in " The Times." She
puts her parcel down, unwraps an apron, half a loaf,
two onions, three potatoes, and a tiny piece of bacon.
Taking a teapot from the cupboard, she rinses it,
shakes into it some powdered tea out of a screw of
paper, puts it on the hearth, and sitting in a wooden
chair quietly begins to cry.

JONES. [*Stirring and yawning.*] That you? What's
the time?

MRS. JONES. [*Drying her eyes, and in her usual voice.*]
Half-past two.

JONES. What you back so soon for?

37

MRS. JONES. I only had the half-day to-day, Jem.

JONES. [*On his back, and in a drowsy voice.*] Got anything for dinner?

MRS. JONES. Mrs. Barthwick's cook gave me a little bit of bacon. I'm going to make a stew. [*She prepares for cooking.*] There's fourteen shillings owing for rent, James, and of course I've only got two and fourpence. They'll be coming for it to-day.

JONES. [*Turning towards her on his elbow.*] Let 'em come and find my surprise packet. I've had enough o' this tryin' for work. Why should I go round and round after a job like a bloomin' squirrel in a cage. " Give us a job, sir "—" Take a man on "—" Got a wife and three children." Sick of it I am! I'd sooner lie here and rot. " Jones, you come and join the demonstration; come and 'old a flag, and listen to the ruddy orators, and go 'ome as empty as you came." There's some that seems to like *that*—the sheep! When I go seekin' for a job now, and see the brutes lookin' me up an' down, it's like a thousand serpents in me. I'm not arskin' for any treat. A man wants to sweat hisself silly and not allowed— that's a rum start, ain't it? A man wants to sweat his soul out to keep the breath in him and ain't allowed—that's justice—that's freedom and all the rest of it . [*He turns his face towards the wall.*] You're so milky mild; you don't know what goes on inside o' me. I'm done with the silly game. If they want me, let 'em come for me !

[MRS. JONES *stops cooking and stands unmoving at the table.*]

I've tried and done with it, I tell you. I've never been afraid of what's before *me*. You mark my words —if you think they've broke my spirit, you're mistook. I'll lie and rot sooner than arsk 'em again. What makes you stand like that—you long-sufferin', Gawd-forsaken image—that's why I can't keep my hands off you. So now you know. Work! You can work, but you haven't the spirit of a louse!

MRS. JONES. [*Quietly.*] You talk more wild some-times when you're yourself, James, than when you're not. If you don't get work, how are we to go on? They won't let us stay here; they're looking to their money to-day, I know.

JONES. I see this Barthwick o' yours every day goin' down to Pawlyment snug and comfortable to talk his silly soul out; an' I see that young calf, his son, swellin' it about, and goin' on the razzle-dazzle. Wot 'ave they done that makes 'em any better than wot I am? They never did a day's work in their lives. I see 'em day after day——

MRS. JONES. And I wish you wouldn't come after me like that, and hang about the house. You don't seem able to keep away at all, and whatever you do it for I can't think, because of course they notice it.

JONES. I suppose I may go where I like. Where *may* I go? The other day I went to a place in the Edgware Road. "Gov'nor," I says to the boss,

"take me on," I says. "I 'aven't done a stroke o'
work not these two months; it takes the heart out
of a man," I says; "I'm one to work; I'm not afraid
of anything you can give me '"　"My good man,"
'e says, "I've had thirty of you here this morning.
I took the first two," he says, "and that's all I want."
"Thank you, then rot the world!" I says. "Blas-
phemin'," he says, "is not the way to get a job.
Out you go, my lad!" [*He laughs sardonically.*] Don't
you raise your voice because you're starvin'; don't yer
even think of it; take it lyin' down! Take it like a
sensible man, carn't you? And a little way down
the street a lady says to me: [*Pinching his voice*]
"D'you want to earn a few pence, my man?" and
gives me her dog to 'old outside a shop—fat as a
butler 'e was—tons o' meat had gone to the makin'
of *him*. It did 'er good, it did, made 'er feel 'erself
that *charitable*, but I see 'er lookin' at the copper
standin' alongside o' me, for fear I should make off
with 'er bloomin' fat dog. [*He sits on the edge of the
bed and puts a boot on. Then looking up.*] What's in
that head o' yours? [*Almost pathetically.*] Carn't you
speak for once?

> [*There is a knock, and* MRS. SEDDON, *the landlady,
> appears, an anxious, harassed, shabby woman
> in working clothes.*

MRS. SEDDON. I thought I 'eard you come in, Mrs.
Jones. I've spoke to my 'usband, but he says he
really can't afford to wait another day.

JONES. [*With scowling jocularity.*] Never you mind

what your 'usband says, you go your own way like a proper independent woman. Here, Jenny, chuck her that.

> [*Producing a sovereign from his trousers pocket, he throws it to his wife, who catches it in her apron with a gasp.* JONES *resumes the lacing of his boots.*

MRS. JONES. [*Rubbing the sovereign stealthily.*] I'm very sorry we're so late with it, and of course it's fourteen shillings, so if you've got six that will be right.

> [MRS. SEDDON *takes the sovereign and fumbles for the change.*

JONES. [*With his eyes fixed on his boots.*] Bit of a surprise for yer, ain't it?

MRS. SEDDON. Thank you, and I'm sure I'm very much obliged. [*She does indeed appear surprised.*] I'll bring you the change.

JONES. [*Mockingly.*] Don't mention it.

MRS. SEDDON. Thank you, and I'm sure I'm very much obliged. [*She slides away.*

> [MRS. JONES *gazes at* JONES, *who is still lacing up his boots.*

JONES. I've had a bit of luck. [*Pulling out the crimson purse and some loose coins.*] Picked up a purse—seven pound and more.

MRS. JONES. Oh, James!

JONES. Oh, James! What about Oh, James! I picked it up I tell you. This is lost property, this is!

MRS. JONES. But isn't there a name in it, or something?

JONES. Name? No, there ain't no name. This don't belong to such as 'ave visitin' cards. This belongs to a perfec' lidy. Tike an' smell it. [*He pitches her the purse, which she puts gently to her nose.*] Now, you tell me what I ought to have done. You tell me that. You can always tell me what I ought to ha' done, can't yer?

MRS. JONES. [*Laying down the purse.*] I can't say what you ought to have done, James. Of course the money wasn't yours; you've taken somebody else's money.

JONES. Finding's keeping. I'll take it as wages for the time I've gone about the streets asking for what's my rights. I'll take it for what's *overdue,* d'ye hear? [*With strange triumph.*] I've got money in my pocket, my girl.

[MRS. JONES *goes on again with the preparation of the meal,* JONES *looking at her furtively.*] Money in my pocket! And I'm not goin' to waste it. With this 'ere money I'm goin' to Canada. I'll let you have a pound. [*A silence.*] You've often talked of leavin' me. You've often told me I treat you badly —well I 'ope you'll be glad when I'm gone.

MRS. JONES. [*Impassively.*] You *have* treated me very badly, James, and of course I can't prevent your going; but I can't tell whether I shall be glad when you're gone.

JONES. It'll change my luck. I've 'ad nothing but

bad luck since I first took up with you. [*More softly.*] And you've 'ad no bloomin' picnic.

MRS. JONES. Of course it would have been better for us if we had never met. We weren't meant for each other. But you're set against me, that's what you are, and you *have* been for a long time. And you treat me so badly, James, going after that Rosie and all. You don't ever seem to think of the children that I've had to bring into the world, and of all the trouble I've had to keep them, and what'll become of them when you're gone.

JONES. [*Crossing the room gloomily.*] If you think I want to leave the little beggars you're bloomin' well mistaken.

MRS. JONES. Of course I know you're fond of them.

JONES. [*Fingering the purse, hal angrily.*] Well, then, you stow it, old girl. The kids'll get along better with you than when I'm here. If I'd ha' known as much as I do now, I'd never ha' had one o' them. What's the use o' bringin' 'em into a state o' things like this? It's a crime, that's what it is; but you find it out too late; that's what's the matter with this 'ere world.

[*He puts the purse back in his pocket.*

MRS. JONES. Of course it would have been better for them, poor little things; but they're your own children, and I wonder at you talkin' like that. I should miss them dreadfully if I was to lose them.

JONES. [*Sullenly.*] An' you ain't the only one. If I make money out there—— [*Looking up, he sees her shaking out his coat—in a changed voice*] Leave that coat alone!

[*The silver box drops from the pocket, scattering
the cigarettes upon the bed. Taking up the
box she stares at it ; he rushes at her and
snatches the box away.*

Mrs. Jones. [*Cowering back against the bed.*] Oh,
Jem ! oh, Jem !

Jones. [*Dropping the box on to the table.*] You mind
what you're sayin' ! When I go out I'll take and
chuck it in the water along with that there purse.
I 'ad it when I was in liquor, and for what you do
when you're in liquor you're not responsible—and
that's Gawd's truth as you ought to know. I don't
want the thing—I won't have it. I took it out o'
spite. I'm no thief, I tell you; and don't you call
me one, or it'll be the worse for you.

Mrs. Jones. [*Twisting her apron strings.*] It's Mr.
Barthwick's ! You've taken away my reputation. Oh,
Jem, whatever made you ?

Jones. What d'you mean ?

Mrs. Jones. It's been missed ; they think it's me.
Oh ! whatever made you do it, Jem ?

Jones. I tell you I was in liquor. I don't want it ;
what's the good of it to me ? If I were to pawn it
they'd only nab me. I'm no thief. I'm no worse
than wot that yonng Barthwick is ; he brought
'ome that purse that I picked up—a lady's purse—
'ad it off 'er in a row, kept sayin' 'e'd scored 'er
off. Well, I scored 'im off. Tight as an owl 'e
was ! And d'you think anything'll happen to
him ?

MRS. JONES. [*As though speaking to herself.*] Oh, Jem! it's the bread out of our mouths!

JONES. Is it then? I'll make it hot for 'em yet. What about that purse? What about young Barthwick?

[MRS. JONES *comes forward to the table and tries to take the box;* JONES *prevents her.*]

What do you want with that? You drop it, I say!

MRS. JONES. I'll take it back and tell them all about it. [*She attempts to wrest the box from him.*

JONES. Ah, would yer?

[*He drops the box, and rushes on her with a snarl. She slips back past the bed. He follows; a chair is overturned. The door is opened;* SNOW *comes in, a detective in plain clothes and bowler hat, with clipped moustaches.* JONES *drops his arms,* MRS. JONES *stands by the window gasping;* SNOW, *advancing swiftly to the table, puts his hand on the silver box.*

SNOW. Doin' a bit o' skylarkin'? Fancy this is what I'm after. J.B., the very same. [*He gets back to the door, scrutinising the crest and cypher on the box. To* MRS. JONES.] I'm a police officer. Are you Mrs. Jones?

MRS. JONES. Yes, sir.

SNOW. My instructions are to take you on a charge of stealing this box from J. Barthwick, Esquire, M.P., of 6, Rockingham Gate. Anything you say may be used against you. Well, missis?

MRS. JONES. [*In her quiet voice, still out of breath, her hand upon her breast.*] Of course I did *not* take it, sir. I never have taken anything that didn't belong to me ; and of course I know nothing about it.

SNOW. You were at the house this morning ; you did the room in which the box was left ; you were alone in the room. I find the box 'ere. You say you didn't take it ?

MRS. JONES. Yes, sir, of course I say I did not take it, because I did *not.*

SNOW. Then how does the box come to be here ?

MRS. JONES. I would rather not say anything about it.

SNOW. Is this your husband ?

MRS. JONES. Yes, sir, this is my husband, sir.

SNOW. Do you wish to say anything before I take her ?

[JONES *remains silent, with his head bent down.*]

Well then, Missis. I'll just trouble you to come along with me quietly.

MRS. JONES. [*Twisting her hands.*] Of course I wouldn't say I hadn't taken it if I had—and I *didn't* take it, indeed I didn't. Of course I know appearances are against me, and I can't tell you what really happened. But my children are at school, and they'll be coming home—and I don't know what they'll do without me !

SNOW. Your 'usband'll see to them, don't you worry. [*He takes the woman gently by the arm.*

JONES. You drop it—she's all right! [*Sullenly.*] I took the thing myself.

SNOW. [*Eyeing him.*] There, there, it does you credit. Come along, Missis.

JONES. [*Passionately.*] Drop it, I say, you blooming teck. She's my wife; she's a respectable woman. Take her if you dare!

SNOW. Now, now. What's the good of this? Keep a civil tongue, and it'll be the better for all of us.

> [*He puts his whistle in his mouth and draws the woman to the door.*

JONES. [*With a rush.*] Drop her, and put up your 'ands, or I'll soon make yer. You leave her alone, will yer! Don't I tell yer, I took the thing myself!

SNOW. [*Blowing his whistle.*] Drop your hands, or I'll take you too.   Ah, would you?

> [JONES, *closing, deals him a blow.   A Policeman in uniform appears ; there is a short struggle and* JONES *is overpowered.*   MRS. JONES *raises her hands and drops her face on them.*
>
> *The curtain falls.*

SCENE II

[*The* BARTHWICKS' *dining-room the same evening.   The* BARTHWICKS *are seated at dessert.*

MRS. BARTHWICK. John! [*A silence broken by the cracking of nuts.*]   John!

D

BARTHWICK. I wish you'd speak about the nuts—they're uneatable.   [*He puts one in his mouth.*

MRS. BARTHWICK. It's not the season for them.   I called on the Holyroods.

[BARTHWICK *fills his glass with port.*

JACK. Crackers, please, dad.

[BARTHWICK *passes the crackers. His demeanour is reflective.*

MRS. BARTHWICK. Lady Holyrood has got very stout.   I've noticed it coming for a long time.

BARTHWICK. [*Gloomily.*] Stout ? [*He takes up the crackers—with transparent airiness.*] The Holyroods had some trouble with their servants, hadn't they ?

JACK. Crackers, please, dad.

BARTHWICK. [*Passing the crackers.*]   It got into the papers.   The cook, wasn't it ?

MRS. BARTHWICK. No, the lady's maid. I was talking it over with Lady Holyrood. The girl used to have her young man to see her.

BARTHWICK. [*Uneasily.*] I'm not sure they were wise——

MRS. BARTHWICK. My dear John, what are you talking about ? How could there be any alternative ? Think of the effect on the other servants !

BARTHWICK. Of course in principle — I wasn't thinking of that.

JACK. [*Maliciously.*] Crackers, please, dad.

[BARTHWICK *is compelled to pass the crackers.*

MRS. BARTHWICK. Lady Holyrood told me : "I had her up," she said; "I said to her, 'You'll leave my house at once ; I think your conduct disgraceful. I can't tell, I don't know, and I don't wish to know, what you were doing. I send you away on principle ; you need not come to me for a character.' And the girl said : ' If you don't give me my notice, my lady, I want a month's wages. I'm perfectly respectable. I've done nothing.' "—Done nothing !

BARTHWICK. H'm !

MRS. BARTHWICK. Servants have too much licence. They hang together so terribly you never can tell what they're really thinking ; it's as if they were all in a conspiracy to keep you in the dark. Even with Marlow, you feel that he never lets you know what's really in his mind. I hate that secretiveness ; it destroys all confidence. I feel sometimes I should like to shake him.

JACK. Marlow's a most decent chap. It's simply beastly every one knowing your affairs.

BARTHWICK. The less you say about that the better !

MRS. BARTHWICK. It goes all through the lower classes. You can *not* tell when they are speaking the truth. To-day when I was shopping after leaving the Holyroods, one of these unemployed came up and spoke to me. I suppose I only had twenty yards or so to walk to the carriage, but he seemed to spring up in the street.

BARTHWICK. Ah ! You must be very careful whom you speak to in these days.

MRS. BARTHWICK. I didn't answer him, of course. But I could see at once that he wasn't telling the truth.

BARTHWICK. [*Cracking a nut.*] There's one very good rule—look at their eyes.

JACK. Crackers, please, Dad.

BARTHWICK. [*Passing the crackers.*] If their eyes are straightforward I sometimes give them sixpence. It's against my principles, but it's most difficult to refuse. If you see that they're desperate, and dull, and shifty-looking, as so many of them are, it's certain to mean drink, or crime, or something unsatisfactory.

MRS. BARTHWICK. This man had dreadful eyes. He looked as if he could commit a murder. "I've 'ad nothing to eat to-day," he said. Just like that.

BARTHWICK. What was William about? He ought to have been waiting.

JACK. [*Raising his wineglass to his nose.*] Is this the '63, Dad?

[BARTHWICK, *holding his wine-glass to his eye, lowers it and passes it before his nose.*

MRS. BARTHWICK. I hate people that can't speak the truth. [*Father and son exchange a look behind their port.*] It's just as easy to speak the truth as not. *I've* always found it easy enough. It makes it impossible to tell what is genuine; one feels as if one were continually being taken in.

BARTHWICK. [*Sententiously.*] The lower classes are their own enemies. If they would only trust us, they would get on so much better.

MRS. BARTHWICK. But even then it's so often their own fault. Look at that Mrs. Jones this morning.

BARTHWICK. I only want to do what's right in that

matter. I had occasion to see Roper this afternoon.
I mentioned it to him. He's coming in this evening.
It all depends on what the detective says. I've had
my doubts. I've been thinking it over.

MRS. BARTHWICK. The woman impressed me most
unfavourably. She seemed to have no shame. That
affair she was talking about——she and the man when
they were young, so immoral! And before you and
Jack! I could have put her out of the room!

BARTHWICK. Oh! I don't want to excuse them,
but in looking at these matters one must consider——

MRS. BARTHWICK. Perhaps you'll say the man's
employer was wrong in dismissing him?

BARTHWICK. Of course not. It's not there that I
feel doubt. What I ask myself is——

JACK. Port, please, Dad.

BARTHWICK. [*Circulating the decanter in religious
imitation of the rising and setting of the sun.*] I ask
myself whether we are sufficiently careful in making
inquiries about people before we engage them,
especially as regards moral conduct.

JACK. Pass the port, please, Mother!

MRS. BARTHWICK. [*Passing it.*] My dear boy, aren't
you drinking too much?

[JACK *fills his glass.*

MARLOW. [*Entering.*] Detective Snow to see you,
sir.

BARTHWICK. [*Uneasily.*] Ah! say I'll be with him
in a minute.

Mrs. Barthwick. [*Without turning.*] Let him come in here, Marlow.

> [Snow *enters in an overcoat, his bowler hat in hand.*

Barthwick. [*Half rising.*] Oh! Good evening!

Snow. Good evening, sir; good evening, ma'am. I've called round to report what I've done, rather late, I'm afraid—another case took me away. [*He takes the silver box out of his pocket, causing a sensation in the* Barthwick *family.*] This is the identical article, I believe.

Barthwick. Certainly, certainly.

Snow. Havin' your crest and cypher, as you described to me, sir, I'd no hesitation in the matter.

Barthwick. Excellent. Will you have a glass of— [*he glances at the waning port*]—er—sherry—[*pours out sherry*]. Jack, just give Mr. Snow this.

> [Jack *rises and gives the glass to* Snow; *then, lolling in his chair, regards him indolently.*

Snow. [*Drinking off wine and putting down the glass.*] After seeing you I went round to this woman's lodgings, sir. It's a low neighbourhood, and I thought it as well to place a constable below—and not without 'e was wanted, as things turned out.

Barthwick. Indeed!

Snow. Yes, sir, I 'ad some trouble. I asked her to account for the presence of the article. She could give me no answer, except to deny the theft; so I took her into custody; then her husband came for me, so I was obliged to take him, too, for assault. He was very violent on the way to the station—very violent —threatened you and your son, and altogether he was a handful, I can tell you.

MRS. BARTHWICK. What a ruffian he must be!

SNOW. Yes, ma'am, a rough customer.

JACK. [*Sipping his wine, bemused.*] Punch the beggar's head.

SNOW. Given to drink, as I understand, Sir.

MRS. BARTHWICK. It's to be hoped he will get a severe punishment.

SNOW. The odd thing is, sir, that he persists in sayin' he took the box himself.

BARTHWICK. Took the box himself! [*He smiles.*] What does he think to gain by that?

SNOW. He says the young gentleman was intoxicated last night—[JACK *stops the cracking of a nut, and looks at Snow.* BARTHWICK, *losing his smile, has put his wineglass down; there is a silence*—SNOW, *looking from face to face, remarks*]—took him into the house and gave him whisky; and under the influence of an empty stomach the man says he took the box.

MRS. BARTHWICK. The impudent wretch!

BARTHWICK. D'you mean that he—er—intends to put this forward to-morrow——

SNOW. That'll be his line, sir; but whether he's endeavouring to shield his wife, or whether [*he looks at* JACK) there's something in it, will be for the magistrate to say.

MRS. BARTHWICK. [*Haughtily.*] Something in what?

much difficulty.   These things are very quick settled.

BARTHWICK. [*Doubtfully.*] You think so—you think so?

JACK. [*Rousing himself.*] I say, what shall I have to swear to?

SNOW. That's best known to yourself, sir. [*Retreating to the door.*] Better employ a solicitor, sir, in case anything should arise. We shall have the butler to prove the loss of the article. You'll excuse me going, I'm rather pressed to-night. The case may come on any time after eleven. Good evening, sir ; good evening, ma'am. I shall have to produce the box in court to-morrow, so if you'll excuse me, sir, I may as well take it with me.

> [*He takes the silver box and leaves them with a little bow.*
>
> [BARTHWICK *makes a move to follow him, then dashing his hands beneath his coat tails, speaks with desperation.*

BARTHWICK. I do wish you'd leave me to manage things myself. You *will* put your nose into matters you know nothing of. A pretty mess you've made of this !

MRS. BARTHWICK. [*Coldly.*] I don't in the least know what you're talking about. If you can't stand up for your rights, I can. I've no patience with your principles, it's such nonsense.

BARTHWICK. Principles ! Good Heavens ! What have principles to do with it for goodness' sake ?

Don't you know that Jack was drunk last night!

JACK. Dad!

MRS. BARTHWICK. [*In horror rising.*] Jack!

JACK. Look here, mother—I had supper. Everybody does. I mean to say—you know what I mean—it's absurd to call it being drunk. At Oxford everybody gets a bit " on " sometimes——

MRS. BARTHWICK. Well I think it's most dreadful! If that is really what you do at Oxford——

JACK. [*Angrily.*] Well, why did you send me there? One must do as other fellows do. It's such nonsense, I mean, to call it being drunk. Of course I'm awfully sorry. I've had such a beastly headache all day.

BARTHWICK. Tcha! If you'd only had the common decency to remember what happened when you came in. Then we should know what truth there was in what this fellow says—as it is, it's all the most confounded darkness

JACK. [*Staring as though at half-formed visions.*] I just get a—and then—it's gone——

MRS. BARTHWICK. Oh, Jack! do you mean to say you were so tipsy you can't even remember——

JACK. Look here, mother! Of course I remember I came—I must have come——

BARTHWICK. [*Unguardedly, and walking up and down.*] Tcha!—and that infernal purse! Good Heavens! It'll get into the papers. Who on earth could have foreseen a thing like this? Better to have lost a dozen cigarette boxes, and said nothing about it. [*To his wife*] It's all your doing. I told you so from the first. I wish to goodness Roper would come!

MRS. BARTHWICK. [*Sharply.*] I don't know what you're talking about, John.

BARTHWICK. [*Turning on her.*] No, you—you—you don't know anything! [*Sharply.*] Where the devil is Roper? If he can see a way out of this he's a better man than I take him for. I defy *anyone* to see a way out of it. *I* can't.

JACK. Look here, don't excite Dad—I can simply say I was too beastly tired, and don't remember anything except that I came in and [*in a dying voice*] went to bed the same as usual.

BARTHWICK. Went to bed? Who knows where you went—I've lost all confidence. For all I know you slept on the floor.

JACK. [*Indignantly.*] I didn't, I slept on the——

BARTHWICK. [*Sitting on the sofa.*] Who cares where you slept; what does it matter if he mentions the —the—a perfect disgrace?

MRS. BARTHWICK. *What?* [*A silence.*] I *insist* on knowing.

JACK. Oh! nothing——

MRS. BARTHWICK. Nothing? What do you mean by nothing, Jack? There's your father in such a state about it——

JACK. It's only my purse.

MRS. BARTHWICK. Your purse! You know perfectly well you haven't got one.

JACK. Well, it was somebody else's—It was all a joke—I didn't want the beastly thing——

MRS. BARTHWICK. Do you mean that you had another person's purse, and that this man took it too?

BARTHWICK. Tcha! Of course he took it too! A man like that Jones will make the most of it. It'll get into the papers.

MRS. BARTHWICK. I don't understand. What on earth is all the fuss about? [*Bending over* JACK, *and softly.*) Jack now, tell me dear! Don't be afraid. What is it? Come!

JACK. Oh, don't mother !

MRS. BARTHWICK. But don't what, dear?

JACK. It was pure sport. I don't know how I got the thing. Of course I'd had a bit of a row—I didn't know what I was doing—I was—I was—well, you know—I suppose I must have pulled the bag out of her hand.

MRS. BARTHWICK. Out of her hand? Whose hand? What bag—whose bag?

JACK. Oh! I don't know—*her* bag—it belonged to —[*in a desperate and rising voice*] a woman.

MRS. BARTHWICK. A woman? *Oh! Jack! No!*

JACK. [*Jumping up.*] You *would* have it. I didn't want to tell you. It's not my fault.

> [*The door opens and* MARLOW *ushers in a man of middle age, inclined to corpulence, in evening dress. He has a ruddy, thin moustache, and dark, quick-moving little eyes. His eyebrows are Chinese.*

MARLOW. Mr. Roper, sir.   [*He leaves the room.*

ROPER. [*With a quick look round.*] How do you do?

[*But neither* JACK *nor* MRS. BARTHWICK *make a sign.*

BARTHWICK. [*Hurrying.*] Thank goodness you've come, Roper. You remember what I told you this afternoon; we've just had the detective here.

ROPER. Got the box?

BARTHWICK. Yes, yes, but look here—it wasn't the charwoman at all ; her drunken loafer of a husband took the things—he says that fellow there [*he waves his hand at* JACK, *who with his shoulder raised, seems trying to ward off a blow*] let him into the house last night. Can you imagine such a thing?

[*Roper laughs.*

BARTHWICK. [*With excited emphasis.*] It's no laughing matter, Roper. I told you about that business of Jack's too—don't you see—the brute took both the things—took that infernal purse. It'll get into the papers.

ROPER. [*Raising his eyebrows.*] H'm ! The purse ! Depravity in high life ! What does your son say ?

BARTHWICK. He remembers nothing. D——n ! Did you ever see such a mess ? It'll get into the papers.

MRS. BARTHWICK. [*With her hand across her eyes.*] No ! it's not that——

[BARTHWICK *and* ROPER *turn and look at her.*

BARTHWICK. It's the idea of that woman—she's just heard——

> [ROPER *nods. And* MRS. BARTHWICK, *setting her lips, gives a slow look at* JACK, *and sits down at the table.*]

What on earth's to be done, Roper? A ruffian like this Jones will make all the capital he can out of that purse.

MRS. BARTHWICK. I don't believe that Jack took that purse.

BARTHWICK. What—when the woman came here for it this morning?

MRS. BARTHWICK. Here? She had the impudence? Why wasn't I told?

> [*She looks round from face to face—no one answers her, there is a pause.*

BARTHWICK. [*Suddenly.*] What's to be done, Roper?

ROPER. [*Quietly to* JACK.] I suppose you didn't leave your latch-key in the door?

JACK. [*Sullenly.*] Yes, I did.

BARTHWICK. Good heavens! What next?

MRS. BARTHWICK. I'm certain you never let that man into the house, Jack, it's a wild invention. I'm sure there's not a word of truth in it, Mr. Roper.

ROPER. [*Very suddenly*]. Where did you sleep last night?

JACK. [*Promptly.*] On the sofa, there—[*hesitating*] that is—I——

BARTHWICK. On the sofa? D'you mean to say you didn't go to bed?

JACK. [*Sullenly*] No.

BARTHWICK. If you don't remember anything, how can you remember that?

JACK. Because I woke up there in the morning.

MRS. BARTHWICK.   Oh, Jack!

BARTHWICK. Good Gracious!

JACK. And Mrs. Jones saw me. I wish you wouldn't bait me so.

ROPER. Do you remember giving any one a drink?

JACK. By Jove, I do seem to remember a fellow with—a fellow with—— [*He looks at Roper.*] I say, d'you want me——?

ROPER. [*Quick as lightning.*]   With a dirty face?

JACK. [*With illumination.*] I do—I distinctly remember his——

> [BARTHWICK *moves abruptly;* MRS. BARTHWICK
> *looks at* ROPER *angrily, and touches her son's
> arm.*

MRS. BARTHWICK. You don't remember, it's ridiculous!   I don't believe the man was ever here at all.

BARTHWICK. You must speak the truth, if it *is* the truth.   But if you *do* remember such a dirty business, I shall wash my hands of you altogether.

JACK. [*Glaring at them.*] Well, what the devil——

MRS. BARTHWICK. Jack!

JACK. Well, mother, I—I don't know what you *do* want.

MRS. BARTHWICK. We want you to speak the truth and say you never let this low man into the house.

BARTHWICK. Of course if you think that you really

gave this man whisky in that disgraceful way, and let him see what you'd been doing, and were in such a disgusting condition that you don't remember a word of it——

ROPER. [*Quick.*] I've no memory myself—never had.

BARTHWICK. [*Desperately.*] I don't know what you're to say.

ROPER [*To* JACK.] Say nothing at all! Don't put yourself in a false position. The man stole the things or the woman stole the things, you had nothing to do with it. You were asleep on the sofa.

MRS. BARTHWICK. Your leaving the latchkey in the door was quite bad enough, there's no need to mention anything else. [*Touching his forehead softly.*] My dear, how hot your head is!

JACK. But I want to know what I'm to do. [*Passionately.*] I won't be badgered like this.

[MRS. BARTHWICK *recoils from him.*

ROPER. [*Very quickly.*] You forget all about it. You were asleep.

JACK. Must I go down to the Court to-morrow?

ROPER. [*Shaking his head.*] No.

BARTHWICK. [*In a relieved voice.*] Is that so?

ROPER. Yes.

BARTHWICK. But *you'll* go, Roper.

ROPER. Yes.

JACK. [*With wan cheerfulness.*] Thanks, awfully! So long as I don't have to go. [*Putting his hand up to his head.*] I think if you'll excuse me—I've had a most beastly day. [*He looks from his father to his mother.*

E

MRS. BARTHWICK. [*Turning quickly.*] Good night, my boy.

JACK. Good-night, mother.

> [*He goes out.*   MRS. BARTHWICK *heaves a sigh.*
> *There is a silence.*

BARTHWICK. He gets off too easily. But for my money that woman would have prosecuted him.

ROPER. You find money useful.

BARTHWICK. I've my doubts whether we ought to hide the truth——

ROPER. There'll be a remand.

BARTHWICK. What ! D'you mean he'll have to *appear* on the remand ?

ROPER. Yes.

BARTHWICK. H'm, I thought you'd be able to—— Look here, Roper, you *must* keep that purse out of the papers.   [ROPER *fixes his little eyes on him and nods.*]

MRS. BARTHWICK. Mr. Roper, don't you think the magistrate ought to be told what sort of people these Joneses are ; I mean about their immorality before they were married.   I don't know if John told you.

ROPER. Afraid it's not material.

MRS. BARTHWICK. Not material ?

ROPER. Purely private life ! May have happened to the magistrate.

BARTHWICK. [*With a movement as if to shift a burden.*] Then you'll take the thing into your hands ?

ROPER. If the gods are kind. [*He holds his hand out.*]

BARTHWICK. [*Shaking it dubiously.*] Kind—eh ? What ? You going ?

ROPER. Yes. I've another case, something like yours—most unexpected.

> [*He bows to* MRS. BARTHWICK *and goes out, followed by* BARTHWICK, *talking to the last.* MRS. BARTHWICK *at the table bursts into smothered sobs.* BARTHWICK *returns.*

BARTHWICK. [*To himself.*] There'll be a scandal.

MRS. BARTHWICK. [*Disguising her grief at once.*] I simply can't imagine what Roper means by making a joke of a thing like that !

BARTHWICK. [*Staring strangely.*] You ! You can't imagine anything ! You've no more imagination than a fly !

MRS. BARTHWICK. [*Angrily.*] You dare to tell me that I have no imagination.

BARTHWICK. [*Flustered.*] I—I'm upset. From beginning to end, the whole thing has been utterly against my principles.

MRS. BARTHWICK. Rubbish ! You haven't any ! Your principles are nothing in the world but sheer—fright !

BARTHWICK. [*Walking to the window.*] I've never been frightened in my life. You heard what Roper said. It's enough to upset any one when a thing like this happens. Everything one says and does seems to turn in one's mouth—it's—it's uncanny. It's not the sort of thing I've been accustomed to. [*As though stifling, he throws the window open. The faint sobbing of a child comes in.*] What's that ?

> [*They listen.*

MRS. BARTHWICK. [*Sharply.*] I can't stand that crying. I must send Marlow to stop it. My nerves are all on edge. [*She rings the bell.*]

BARTHWICK. I'll shut the window; you'll hear nothing. [*He shuts the window. There is silence.*]

MRS. BARTHWICK. [*Sharply.*] That's no good! It's on my nerves. Nothing upsets me like a child's crying. [MARLOW *comes in.*] What's that noise of crying, Marlow? It sounds like a child.

BARTHWICK. It is a child. I can see it against the railings.

MARLOW. [*Opening the window, and looking out— quietly.*] It's Mrs. Jones's little boy, ma'am; he came here after his mother.

MRS. BARTHWICK. [*Moving quickly to the window.*] Poor little chap! John, we oughtn't to go on with this!

BARTHWICK. [*Sitting heavily in a chair.*] Ah! but it's out of our hands!

> [MRS. BARTHWICK *turns her back to the window. There is an expression of distress on her face. She stands motionless, compressing her lips. The crying begins again.* BARTHWICK *covers his ears with his hands, and* MARLOW *shuts the window. The crying ceases.*
>
> *The curtain falls.*

ACT III

*Eight days have passed, and the scene is a London Police
  Court at one o'clock.   A canopied seat of Justice is
  surmounted by the lion and unicorn.   Before the
  fire a worn-looking* MAGISTRATE *is warming his
  coat-tails, and staring at two little girls in faded blue
  and orange rags, who are placed before the dock.
  Close to the witness-box is a* RELIEVING OFFICER *in
  an overcoat, and a short brown beard.   Beside the little
  girls stands a bald* POLICE CONSTABLE.   *On the front
  bench are sitting* BARTHWICK *and* ROPER, *and behind
  them* JACK.   *In the railed enclosure are seedy-looking
  men and women.   Some prosperous constables sit or
  stand about.*

MAGISTRATE. [*In his paternal and ferocious voice, hissing
his s's.*]   Now let us dispose of these young ladies.

USHER.   Theresa Livens, Maud Livens.

> [*The bald* CONSTABLE *indicates the little girls
>   who remain silent, disillusioned, inattentive.*

Relieving Officer !

> [*The* RELIEVING OFFICER *steps into the witness-box*

USHER.   The evidence you give to the Court shall
be the truth, the whole truth, and nothing but the
truth, so help you God !   Kiss the book !

> [*The book is kissed.*

RELIEVING OFFICER. [*In a monotone, pausing slightly at each sentence end, that his evidence may be inscribed.*] About ten o'clock this morning, your Worship, I found these two little girls in Blue Street, Pulham, crying outside a public-house. Asked where their home was, they said they had no home. Mother had gone away. Asked about their father. Their father had no work. Asked where they slept last night. At their aunt's. I've made inquiries, your Worship. The wife has broken up the home and gone on the streets. The husband is out of work and living in common lodging-houses. The husband's sister has eight children of her own, and says she can't afford to keep these little girls any longer.

MAGISTRATE. [*Returning to his seat beneath the canopy of Justice.*] Now, let me see. You say the mother is on the streets ; what evidence have you of that ?

RELIEVING OFFICER. I have the husband here, your Worship.

MAGISTRATE. Very well ; then let us see him.

    [*There are cries of "* LIVENS.*" The* MAGISTRATE
        leans forward, and stares with hard compas-
        sion at the little girls. LIVENS *comes in. He*
        is quiet, with grizzled hair, and a muffler for
        a collar. He stands beside the witness-box.]
And you are their father ? Now, why don't you keep your little girls at home. How is it you leave them to wander about the streets like this ?

LIVENS. I've got no home, your Worship. I'm

living from 'and to mouth.   I've got no work ; and
nothin' to keep them on.

MAGISTRATE. How is that ?

LIVENS. [*Ashamedly.*]   My wife, she broke my 'ome
up, and pawned the things.

MAGISTRATE. But what made you let her ?

LEVINS. Your Worship, I'd no chance to stop 'er ;
she did it when I was out lookin' for work.

MAGISTRATE. Did you ill-treat her ?

LIVENS. [*Emphatically.*]   I never raised my 'and to
her in my life, your Worship.

MAGISTRATE. Then what was it—did she drink ?

LIVENS. Yes, your Worship.

MAGISTRATE. Was she loose in her behaviour ?

LIVENS. [*In a low voice.*]   Yes, your Worship.

MAGISTRATE. And where is she now ?

LIVENS. I don't know, your Worship.   She went off
with a man, and after that I——

MAGISTRATE. Yes, yes.   Who knows anything of
her ? [*To the bald* CONSTABLE.]   Is she known here ?

RELIEVING OFFICER. Not in this district, your
Worship ; but I have ascertained that she is well
known——

MAGISTRATE. Yes—yes ; we'll stop at that.   Now
[*To the Father*] you say that she has broken up your
home, and left these little girls.   What provision
can you make for them ?   You look a strong man.

LIVENS. So I am, your Worship.   I'm willin'
enough to work, but for the life of me I can't get
anything to do.

MAGISTRATE. But have you tried?

LIVENS. I've tried everything, your Worship—I've tried my 'ardest.

MAGISTRATE. Well, well——   [*There is a silence.*

RELIEVING OFFICER. If your Worship thinks it's a case, my people are willing to take them.

MAGISTRATE. Yes, yes, I know; but I've no evidence that this man is not the proper guardian for his children.   [*He rises and goes back to the fire.*

RELIEVING OFFICER. The mother, your Worship, is able to get access to them.

MAGISTRATE. Yes, yes; the mother, of course, is an improper person to have anything to do with them. [*To the Father.*]   Well, now what do you say?

LIVENS. Your Worship, I can only say that if I could get work I should be only too willing to provide for them.   But what can I do, your Worship? Here I am obliged to live from 'and to mouth in these 'ere common lodging-houses. I'm a strong man—I'm willing to work—I'm half as alive again as some of 'em—but you see, your Worship, my 'air's turned a bit, owing to the fever—[*Touches his hair*]— and that's against me; and I don't seem to get a chance anyhow.

MAGISTRATE. Yes—yes. [*Slowly.*]   Well, I think it's a case. [*Staring his hardest at the little girls.*] Now, are you willing that these little girls should be sent to a home?

LIVENS. Yes, your Worship, I should be very willing.

MAGISTRATE. Well, I'll remand them for a week. Bring them again to-day week; if I see no reason against it then, I'll make an order.

RELIEVING OFFICER. To-day week, your Worship.

> [*The bald* CONSTABLE *takes the little girls out by the shoulders. The Father follows them. The* MAGISTRATE, *returning to his seat, bends over and talks to his* CLERK *inaudibly.*

BARTHWICK. [*Speaking behind his hand.*] A painful case, Roper; very distressing state of things.

ROPER. Hundreds like this in the Police Courts.

BARTHWICK. Most distressing! The more I see of it, the more important this question of the condition of the people seems to become. I shall certainly make a point of taking up the cudgels in the House. I shall move——

> [*The* MAGISTRATE *ceases talking to his* CLERK.

CLERK. Remands.

> BARTHWICK *stops abruptly. There is a stir and* MRS. JONES *comes in by the public door;* JONES, *ushered by policemen, comes from the prisoner's door. They file into the dock.*

CLERK. James Jones, Jane Jones.

USHER. Jane Jones.

BARTHWICK. [*In a whisper.*] The purse—the purse *must* be kept out of it, Roper. Whatever happens you must keep that out of the papers.

> [ROPER *nods.*

BALD CONSTABLE. Hush!

> [MRS. JONES, *dressed in her thin, black, wispy dress, and black straw hat, stands motionless with hands crossed on the front rail of the dock.* JONES *leans against the back rail of the dock, and keeps half turning, glancing defiantly about him. He is haggard and unshaven.*

CLERK. [*Consulting with his papers.*] This is the case remanded from last Wednesday, sir. Theft of a silver cigarette box and assault on the police; the two charges were taken together. Jane Jones! James Jones!

MAGISTRATE. [*Staring.*] Yes, yes; I remember.

CLERK. Jane Jones.

MRS. JONES. Yes, sir.

CLERK. Do you admit stealing a silver cigarette box valued at five pounds, ten shillings, from the house of John Barthwick, M.P., between the hours of 11 P.M. on Easter Monday and 8.45 A.M. on Easter Tuesday last? Yes or no?

MRS. JONES. [*In a low voice.*] No, sir, I do not, sir.

CLERK. James Jones? Do you admit stealing a silver cigarette box valued at five pounds, ten shillings, from the house of John Barthwick, M.P., between the hours of 11 P.M. on Easter Monday and 8.45 A.M. on Easter Tuesday last. And further making an assault on the police when in the execution of their duty at 3 P.M. on Easter Tuesday? Yes or no?

JONES. [*Sullenly.*] Yes, but I've a lot to say about it.

MAGISTRATE. [*To the* CLERK.] Yes—yes. But how comes it that these two people are charged with the same offence? Are they husband and wife?

CLERK. Yes, sir. You remember you ordered a remand for further evidence as to the story of the male prisoner.

MAGISTRATE. Have they been in custody since?

CLERK. You released the woman on her own recognizances, sir.

MAGISTRATE. Yes, yes, this is the case of the silver box; I remember now. Well?

CLERK. Thomas Marlow.

[*The cry of* "THOMAS MARLOW" *is repeated.*
MARLOW *comes in, and steps into the witness-box, and is sworn. The silver box is handed up, and placed on the rail.*

CLERK. [*Reading from his papers.*] Your name is Thomas Marlow? Are you butler to John Barthwick, M.P., of 6, Rockingham Gate?

MARLOW. Yes, sir.

CLERK. Did you between 10.45 and 11 o'clock on the night of Easter Monday last place a silver cigarette box on a tray on the dining-room table at 6, Rockingham Gate? Is that the box?

MARLOW. Yes, sir.

CLERK. And did you miss the same at 8.45 on the following morning, on going to remove the tray?

MARLOW. Yes, sir.

CLERK. Is the female prisoner known to you?

[MARLOW *nods.*]

Is she the charwoman employed at 6, Rockingham Gate? [*Again* MARLOW *nods.*]

Did you at the time of your missing the box find her in the room alone?

MARLOW. Yes, sir.

CLERK. Did you afterwards communicate the loss to your employer, and did he send you to the police station?

MARLOW. Yes, sir.

CLERK. [*To* MRS. JONES.] Have you anything to ask him?

MRS. JONES. No, sir, nothing, thank you, sir.

CLERK. [*To* JONES.] James Jones, have you anything to ask this witness?

JONES. I don't know 'im.

MAGISTRATE. Are you sure you put the box in the place you say at the time you say?

MARLOW. Yes, your Worship.

MAGISTRATE. Very well; then now let us have the officer.

[MARLOW *leaves the box, and* SNOW *goes into it.*

USHER. The evidence you give to the court shall be the truth, the whole truth, and nothing but the truth, so help you God. [*The book is kissed.*

CLERK. [*Reading from his papers.*] Your name is Robert Snow? You are a detective in the X. B. division of the Metropolitan police force? According to instructions received did you on Easter Tuesday last proceed to the prisoner's lodgings at 34, Merthyr Street, St. Soames'? And did you on entering see the box produced, lying on the table?

SNOW. Yes, sir.

CLERK. Is that the box?

SNOW. [*Fingering the box.*] Yes, sir.

CLERK. And did you thereupon take possession of it, and charge the female prisoner with theft of the box from 6, Rockingham Gate? And did she deny the same?

SNOW. Yes, sir.

CLERK. Did you take her into custody?

SNOW. Yes, sir.

MAGISTRATE. What was her behaviour?

SNOW. Perfectly quiet, your Worship. She persisted in the denial. That's all.

MAGISTRATE. Do you know her?

SNOW. No, your Worship.

MAGISTRATE. Is she known here?

BALD CONSTABLE. No, your Worship, they're neither of them known, we've nothing against them at all.

CLERK. [*To* MRS. JONES.] Have you anything to ask the officer?

MRS. JONES. No, sir, thank you, I've nothing to ask him.

MAGISTRATE. Very well then—go on.

CLERK. [*Reading from his papers.*] And while you were taking the female prisoner did the male prisoner interpose, and endeavour to hinder you in the execution of your duty, and did he strike you a blow?

SNOW. Yes, sir.

CLERK. And did he say, "You let her go, I took the box myself"?

SNOW. He did.

CLERK. And did you blow your whistle and obtain the assistance of another constable, and take him into custody?

SNOW. I did.

CLERK. Was he violent on the way to the station, and did he use bad language, and did he several times repeat that he had taken the box himself?

[SNOW *nods.*]

Did you thereupon ask him in what manner he had stolen the box? And did you understand him to say that he had entered the house at the invitation of young Mr. Barthwick

[BARTHWICK, *turning in his seat, frowns at* ROPER.]

after midnight on Easter Monday, and partaken of whisky, and that under the influence of the whisky he had taken the box?

SNOW. I did, sir.

CLERK. And was his demeanour throughout very violent?

SNOW. It *was* very violent.

JONES. [*Breaking in.*] Violent—of course it was. You put your 'ands on my wife when I kept tellin' you I took the thing myself.

MAGISTRATE. [*Hissing, with protruded neck.*] Now—
you will have your chance of saying what you want
to say presently. Have you anything to ask the
officer?

JONES. [*Sullenly.*] No

MAGISTRATE. Very well then. Now let us hear
what the female prisoner has to say first.

MRS. JONES. Well, your Worship, of course I can
only say what I've said all along, that I didn't take
the box.

MAGISTRATE. Yes, but did you know that it was
taken?

MRS. JONES. No, your Worship. And, of course, as
to what my husband says, your Worship, I can't
speak of my own knowledge. Of course, I know
that he came home very late on the Monday night.
It was past one o'clock when he came in, and he was
not himself at all.

MAGISTRATE. Had he been drinking?

MRS. JONES. Yes, your Worship.

MAGISTRATE. And was he drunk?

MRS. JONES. Yes, your Worship, he was almost
quite drunk.

MAGISTRATE And did he say anything to you?

MRS. JONES. No, your Worship, only to call me
names. And of course in the morning when I got
up and went to work he was asleep. And I don't
know anything more about it until I came home
again. Except that Mr. Barthwick—that's my employer, **your** Worship—told me the box was missing.

MAGISTRATE. Yes, yes.

MRS. JONES. But of course when I was shaking out my husband's coat the cigarette-box fell out and all the cigarettes were scattered on the bed.

MAGISTRATE. You say all the cigarettes were scattered on the bed? [*To* SNOW.] Did you see the cigarettes scattered on the bed?

SNOW. No, your Worship, I did not.

MAGISTRATE. You see he says he didn't see them.

JONES. Well, they were there for all that.

SNOW. I can't say, your Worship, that I had the opportunity of going round the room; I had all my work cut out with the male prisoner.

MAGISTRATE. [*To* MRS. JONES.] Well, what more have you to say?

MRS. JONES. Of course when I saw the box, your Worship, I was dreadfully upset, and I couldn't think why he had done such a thing; when the officer came we were having words about it, because it is ruin to me, your Worship, in my profession, and I have three little children dependent on me.

MAGISTRATE. [*Protruding his neck.*] Yes—yes—but what did he say to you?

MRS. JONES. I asked him whatever came over him to do such a thing—and he said it was the drink. He said that he had had too much to drink, and something came over him. And of course, your Worship he had had very little to eat all day, and the drink does go to the head when you have not had enough to eat. Your Worship may not know, but it is the truth.   And I would like to say that all through his married life I have never known him to do such a thing before, though we have passed through great hardships and [*speaking with soft emphasis*] I am quite sure he would not have done it if he had been himself at the time.

MAGISTRATE. Yes, yes.   But don't you know that that is no excuse?

MRS. JONES. Yes, your Worship.   I know that it is no excuse.

> [*The* MAGISTRATE *leans over and parleys with his* CLERK.

JACK. [*Leaning over from his seat behind.*] I say, Dad——

BARTHWICK. Tsst! [*Sheltering his mouth he speaks to* ROPER.] Roper, you had better get up now and say that considering the circumstances and the poverty of the prisoners, we have no wish to proceed any further, and if the magistrate would deal with the case as one of disorder only on the part of——

BALD CONSTABLE. Hssshh!

> [ROPER *shakes his head.*

MAGISTRATE. Now, supposing what you say and what your husband says is true, what I have to consider is—how did he obtain access to this house, and were you in any way a party to his obtaining access? You are the charwoman employed at the house?

MRS. JONES. Yes, your Worship, and of course if I had let him into the house it would have been very

F

wrong of me ; and I have never done such a thing in any of the houses where I have been employed.

MAGISTRATE. Well—so you say.   Now let us hear what story the male prisoner makes of it.

JONES. [*Who leans with his arms on the dock behind, speaks in a slow, sullen voice.*] Wot I say is wot my wife says.   I've never been 'ad up in a police-court before, an' I can prove I took it when in liquor.   I told her, an' she can tell you the same, that I was goin' to throw the thing into the water sooner then 'ave it on my mind.

MAGISTRATE. But how did you get into the *house* ?

JONES. I was passin.'   I was goin' 'ome from the "Goat and Bells."

MAGISTRATE. The "Goat and Bells,"—what is that ?   A public-house ?

JONES. Yes, at the corner.   It was Bank 'oliday, an' I'd 'ad a drop to drink.   I see this young Mr. Barthwick tryin' to find the keyhole on the wrong side of the door.

MAGISTRATE. Well ?

JONES. [*Slowly and with many pauses.*] Well—I 'elped 'im to find it—drunk as a lord 'e was.   He goes on, an' comes back again, and says, I've got nothin' for you, 'e says, but come in an' 'ave a drink.   So I went in just as you might 'ave done yourself.   We 'ad a drink o' whisky just as you might have 'ad, 'nd young Mr. Barthwick says to me, "Take a drink 'nd a smoke.   Take anything you like, 'e says.   And then he went to sleep on the sofa.   I 'ad some more whisky—an' I 'ad a smoke—and I 'ad some more whisky—an' I carn't tell yer what 'appened after that.

MAGISTRATE. Do you mean to say you were so drunk that you can remember nothing?

JACK. [*Softly to his father.*] I say, that's exactly what——

BARTHWICK. Tssh!

JONES. That's what I do mean.

MAGISTRATE. And yet you say you stole the box?

JONES. I never stole the box. I took it.

MAGISTRATE. [*Hissing, with protruded neck.*] You did not steal it—you took it. Did it belong to you— what is that but stealing?

JONES. I took it.

MAGISTRATE. You took it—you took it away from their house and you took it to your house——

JONES. [*Sullenly breaking in.*] I ain't got a house.

MAGISTRATE. Very well, let us hear what this young man Mr.—Mr. Barthwick—has to say to your story.

> [SNOW *leaves the witness-box.   The* BALD CON-
> STABLE *beckons* JACK, *who, clutching his hat,
> goes into the witness-box.* ROPER *moves to
> the table set apart for his profession.*

SWEARING CLERK. The evidence you give to the Court shall be the truth, the whole truth, and nothing but the truth, so help you God.   Kiss the book.

> [*The Book is kissed.*

ROPER. [*Examining.*] What is your name?

F*

JACK [*In a low voice.*] John Barthwick, Junior.

[*The* CLERK *writes it down.*

ROPER. Where do you live ?

JACK. At 6, Rockingham Gate.

[*All his answers are recorded by the Clerk.*

ROPER. You are the son of the owner ?

JACK. [*In a very low voice.*] Yes.

ROPER. Speak up, please. Do you know the prisoner ?

JACK. [*Looking at the* JONESES, *in a low voice.*] I've seen Mrs. Jones. I—[*in a loud voice*] don't know the man.

JONES. Well, I know you !

BALD CONSTABLE. Hssh !

ROPER. Now, did you come in late on the night of Easter Monday ?

JACK. Yes.

ROPER. And did you by mistake leave your latch-key in the door ?

JACK. Yes.

MAGISTRATE. Oh! You left your latchkey in the door ?

ROPER. And is that all you can remember about your coming in ?

JACK. [*In a loud voice.*] Yes, it is.

MAGISTRATE. Now, you have heard the male prisoner s story, what do you say to that ?

JACK. [*Turning to the* MAGISTRATE, *speaks suddenly in a confident, straightforward voice.*] The fact of the matter is, sir, that I'd been out to the theatre that night, and had supper afterwards, and I came in late.

MAGISTRATE. Do you remember this man being outside when you came in?

JACK. No, sir. [*He hesitates.*] I don't think I do.

MAGISTRATE. [*Somewhat puzzled.*] Well, did he help you to open the door, as he says? Did *any* one help you to open the door?

JACK. No, sir—I don't think so, sir—I don't know.

MAGISTRATE. You don't know? But you must know. It isn't a usual thing for you to have the door opened for you, is it?

JACK. [*With a shamefaced smile.*] No.

MAGISTRATE. Very well, then——

JACK. [*Desperately.*] The fact of the matter is, sir, I'm afraid I'd had too much champagne that night.

MAGISTRATE. [*Smiling.*] Oh! you'd had too much champagne?

JONES. May I ask the gentleman a question?

MAGISTRATE. Yes—yes—you may ask him what questions you like.

JONES. Don't you remember you said you was a Liberal, same as your father, and you asked me wot I was?

JACK. [*With his hand against his brow.*] I seem to remember——

JONES. And I said to you, " I'm a bloomin' Conserva*tive*," I said ; an' you said to me, "You look more like one of these 'ere Socialists. Take wotever you like," you said.

JACK. [*With sudden resolution.*] No, I don't.   I
don't remember anything of the sort.

JONES. Well, I do, an' my word's as good as yours.
I've never been had up in a police court before.
Look 'ere, don't you remember you had a sky-blue
bag in your 'and——   [BARTHWICK *jumps.*

ROPER. I submit to your worship that these questions are hardly to the point, the prisoner having
admitted that he himself does not remember anything. [*There is a smile on the face of Justice.*] It is a
case of the blind leading the blind.

JONES. [*Violently.*] I've done no more than wot he
'as. I'm a poor man   I've got no money an' no
friends—he's a toff—he can do wot I can't.

MAGISTRATE. Now, now !   All this won't help you
—you must be quiet.   You say you took this box ?
Now, what made you take it ?   Were you pressed
for money ?

JONES. I'm always pressed for money.

MAGISTRATE. Was that the reason you took it ?
JONES. No.

MAGISTRATE. [*To* SNOW.] Was anything found on
him ?

SNOW. Yes, your worship.   There was six pounds
twelve shillin's found on him, and this purse.

> [*The red silk purse is handed to the* MAGIS-
> TRATE.   BARTHWICK *rises in his seat, but
> hastily sits down again.*

MAGISTRATE. [*Staring at the purse.*] Yes, yes—let
me see——   [*There is a silence.*]   No, no, I've nothing

before me as to the purse. How did you come by all that money ?

JONES. [*After a long pause, suddenly.*] I declines to say.

MAGISTRATE. But if you had all that money, what made you take this box ?

JONES. I took it out of spite.

MAGISTRATE. [*Hissing, with protruded neck.*] You took it out of spite ? Well now, that's something ! But do you imagine you can go about the town taking things out of spite ?

JONES. If you had my life, if you'd been out of work——

MAGISTRATE. Yes, yes; I know—because you're out of work you think it's an excuse for everything.

JONES. [*Pointing at* JACK.] You ask 'im wot made 'im take the——

ROPER. [*Quietly.*] Does your worship require this witness in the box any longer ?

MAGISTRATE. [*Ironically.*] I think not; he is hardly profitable.

> [JACK *leaves the witness-box, and, hanging his head, resumes his seat.*]

JONES. You ask 'im wot made 'im take the lady's——

> [*But the* BALD CONSTABLE *catches him by the sleeve.*]

BALD CONSTABLE. Sssh !

MAGISTRATE. [*Emphatically.*] Now listen to me.

I've nothing to do with what he may or may not have taken. Why did you resist the police in the execution of their duty?

JONES. It warn't their duty to take my wife, a respectable woman, that 'adn't done nothing.

MAGISTRATE. But I say it was. What made you strike the officer a blow?

JONES. Any man would a struck 'im a blow. I'd strike 'im again, I would.

MAGISTRATE. You are not making your case any better by violence. How do you suppose we could get on if everybody behaved like you?

JONES. [Leaning forward, earnestly.] Well, wot about 'er; who's to make up to 'er for this? Who's to give 'er back 'er good name?

MRS. JONES. Your Worship, it's the children that's preying on his mind, because of course I've lost my work. And I've had to find another room owing to the scandal.

MAGISTRATE. Yes, yes, I know—but if he hadn't acted like this nobody would have suffered.

JONES. [Glaring round at JACK.] I've done no worse than wot 'e 'as. Wot I want to know is wot's goin' to be done to 'im.

[The BALD CONSTABLE again says "Hssh!"

ROPER. Mr. Barthwick wishes it known, your Worship, that considering the poverty of the prisoners he does not press the charge as to the box. Perhaps your Worship would deal with the case as one of disorder

JONES. I don't want it smothered up, I want it all dealt with fair—I want my rights—

MAGISTRATE. [*Rapping his desk.*] Now you have said all you have to say, and you will be quiet.

> [*There is a silence ; the* MAGISTRATE *bends over and parleys with his* CLERK.

Yes, I think I may discharge the woman. [*In a kindly voice he addresses* MRS. JONES, *who stands unmoving with her hands crossed on the rail.*] It is very unfortunate for you that this man has behaved as he has. It is not the consequences to him but the consequences to you. You have been brought here twice, you have lost your work—[*He glares at* JONES] and this is what always happens. Now you may go away, and I am very sorry it was necessary to bring you here at all.

MRS. JONES. [*Softly.*] Thank you very much, your Worship.

> [*She leaves the dock, and looking back at* JONES, *twists her fingers and is still.*

MAGISTRATE. Yes, yes, but I can't pass it over Go away, there's a good woman.

> [MRS. JONES *stands back. The* MAGISTRATE *leans his head on his hand : then raising it he speaks to* JONES.]

Now, listen to me. Do you wish the case to be settled here, or do you wish it to go before a Jury?

JONES. [*Muttering.*] I don't want no Jury.

MAGISTRATE. Very well then, I will deal with it

here. [*After a pause.*] You have pleaded guilty to stealing this Box—

JONES. Not to stealin'—

BALD CONSTABLE. Hssshh

MAGISTRATE. And to assaulting the police——

JONES. Any man as was a man——

MAGISTRATE. Your conduct here has been most improper. You give the excuse that you were drunk when you stole the box. I tell you that is no excuse. If you choose to get drunk and break the law afterwards you must take the consequences. And let me tell you that men like you, who get drunk and give way to your spite or whatever it is that's in you, are—are—a *nuisance to the community.*

JACK. [*Leaning from his seat.*] Dad ' that's what you said to me ?

BARTHWICK. Tsst .

> [*There is a silence, while the* MAGISTRATE *consults his* CLERK ; JONES *leans forward waiting.*

MAGISTRATE. This is your first offence, and I am going to give you a light sentence. [*Speaking sharply, but without expression.*] One month with hard labour.

> [*He bends, and parleys with his* CLERK. *The* BALD CONSTABLE *and another help* JONES *from the dock.*

JONES. [*Stopping and twisting round.*] Call this justice ? What about 'im ? 'E got drunk ! 'E took the purse—'e took the purse but [*in a muffled shout*] it's '*is money got 'im* off—*Justice !*

> [*The prisoner's door is shut on* JONES, *and from the seedy-looking men and women comes a hoarse and whispering groan.*

MAGISTRATE. We will now adjourn for lunch ! [*He rises from his seat.*]

> [*The Court is in a stir.* ROPER *gets up and speaks to the reporter.* JACK, *throwing up his head, walks with a swagger to the corridor;* BARTHWICK *follows.*

MRS. JONES. [*Turning to him with a humble gesture.* Oh ! Sir !—

> [BARTHWICK *hesitates, then yielding to his nerves, he makes a shame-faced gesture of refusal, and hurries out of Court.* MRS. JONES *stands looking after him.*

> *The curtain falls.*